Community Health Centers

Critical Issues in Health and Medicine

Edited by Rima D. Apple, University of Wisconsin–Madison,
and Janet Golden, Rutgers University, Camden

Growing criticism of the U.S. health care system is coming from consumers, politicians, the media, activists, and health care professionals. Critical Issues in Health and Medicine is a collection of books that explores these contemporary dilemmas from a variety of perspectives, among them political, legal, historical, sociological, and comparative, and with attention to crucial dimensions such as race, gender, ethnicity, sexuality, and culture.

Community Health Centers

A Movement and the People
Who Made It Happen

Bonnie Lefkowitz

Rutgers University Press

New Brunswick, New Jersey, and London

Library of Congress Cataloging-in-Publication Data

Lefkowitz, Bonnie.
  Community health centers : a movement and the people who made it happen / Bonnie Lefkowitz.
    p. ; cm. — (Critical issues in health and medicine)
  Includes bibliographical references and index.
  ISBN-13: 978–0–8135–3911–9 (hardcover : alk. paper)
  ISBN-13: 978–0–8135–3912–6 (pbk. : alk. paper)
  1. Community health services—United States—History. I. Title. II. Series.
  [DNLM: 1. Community Health Centers—history—United States. 2. Civil Rights—history—United States. 3. Health Care Reform—history—United States. 4. Health Policy—history—United States. WA 11 AA1 L493c 2007]
  RA445.L38 2007
  362.12—dc22   2006011530

A British Cataloging-in-Publication record for this book is available from the British Library.

Manufactured in the United States of America

Contents

Preface

This book is about a groundbreaking approach to health, a program that by all rights should never have survived, and people with rare foresight and commitment. For forty years or more, men and women have been working in the tenements of New York, the *colonias* of Texas, the working-class neighborhoods of Boston, and the dirt farms of the Deep South to heal the bodies and souls of the disenfranchised through health centers combining primary and preventive care, environmental services, economic development, and empowerment.

Heir to a time of staggering courage, they share a common heritage in the broader movements for civil rights and social justice of the early 1960s. Think what it took for the first civil rights activists to conquer their fear, walk out the door, cross to the white side of the street, and take the first hesitant steps toward freedom. Or for migrant workers in a strange land to leave their jobs in the field and join the fight to humanize a brutal industry.

Many of those who marched, picketed, sat in, registered voters, and went to jail continued to organize in their communities around health care issues. They convinced others to join them and mentored younger people who worked beside them. And they taught countless people who, like me, read about them, visited with them, and were sustained by their example for years to come.

Their work has lasted despite cynicism and inertia, a far more complex and sophisticated opposition to racial equality, the blurring of right and wrong—and sometimes their own feet of clay. It is testimony to the difference one person can make, and to the social contract that many have forgotten.

There are also important lessons for how we provide health care at a time when there are huge discrepancies in access, intractable and even widening disparities in outcomes, and a lack of attention to the things that make us sick in the first place. Today's debates on the public's health are overwhelmed by a preoccupation with genomic advances and market innovations. In contrast, the early centers had a commonsense, holistic philosophy that came from understanding that good health is close to impossible if you have to choose among food, rent, and medicine. If people were hungry, health centers provided food first, then organized cooperatives and helped with employment. If sanitation was lacking, they dug privies and delivered barrels of pure water, and then campaigned for better county services. If people didn't show up, they sent buses and boats; set up shop in fields, shelters, and mobile clinics; and trained community workers in outreach and education. The centers were governed by the people who used them, and brought power where none seemed to exist.

Soon after I joined the national staff of the health center program in 1983, I was called to a meeting with the director, an activist physician turned hard-driving manager. I went, forewarned and armed with calculator and a stack of computer printouts.

"I see you've got your tools," my new boss said approvingly. He had hired me from a policy office close to the seat of power, known for its quantitative skills and penchant for working long hours. I smiled, knowing that my decision to take the health center job was based more on the chance to work with people whose sense of purpose I admired.

I continued to use those technical tools and to ply the trade of a bureaucrat for the next sixteen years, learning both good and bad along the way. The best times were spent visiting the men and women who ran health centers in poor urban neighborhoods and isolated rural areas. Some seemed to exemplify the very idea of community. They knew each street corner or country road, and they showed them to me lovingly, if not always proudly. They knew the people in the tenements and tarpaper shacks, often by name, and understood their problems and their potential. I got enough glimpses of why my hosts were there in the first place to make me hunger for more.

Today my tools are a six-by-nine-inch spiral notebook and a ballpoint pen; sometimes a cassette recorder and a point-and-shoot camera. I set out to record the contributions of these community leaders, to help preserve a legacy of hope and redemption, to extract lessons for the future, and to repay, in small part, those who taught and inspired me.

This is not a scientific study—not even a purposive sample. The 900-plus health centers in every state and several territories include remarkable organizations with outstanding leaders, some that do well but lack that certain spark, and some bad apples. I chose to visit organizations whose leaders had impressed me over the years, narrowing an original list of over twenty to those whose history I could trace from the early days on through to the present. I also tried to be geographically and demographically diverse, although by no means representative of the whole.

Once I decided to visit a place, I was determined to tell the truth about it, warts and all, drawing on an ever-increasing circle of informants to suggest people who remembered the old days, local sources and archived documents. I knew that there had been tensions within the health center family, and struggles with established institutions. Survival has sometimes been costly, as centers dealt with political opposition, cuts in the non-medical services that made them unique in the first place, and the need to compete in a managed care market. But there are also monumental achievements: hard-wrought partnerships, heartwarming reconciliations, thousands of young men and women trained as professionals, and full inclusion of poor people and minorities in the power structure, often for the first time. Most important, patients have been treated with respect and humanity, costly and invasive procedures avoided, racial/ethnic and income disparities reduced, and lives saved—all while the centers have grown exponentially in size and sophistication and made their way in an increasingly complex environment.

I also drew on the knowledge of scores of national leaders—those who developed the first health centers, government officials who funded them and coaxed a growing network into existence, academics who studied them, politicians who determined their fate, and advocates who met the many challenges faced by an antiestablishment program. Some of them are still in the thick of health center affairs. Others have gone on to different things—physicians and center directors to hospitals and managed care plans, professors to new fields of research, elected officials to broader issues. But for every one of them, the health center experience remains central. After all, who else calls their program a movement?

The more I learned, the more I realized that this story touched nearly every part of my life, not just the sixteen years I spent working directly with the centers. Early in my research I discovered that a clinic established by civil rights workers in Mississippi, predecessor to the first fully comprehensive health center, was named for Irving Winik, my family physician when I was growing up in Washington, D.C. It actually operated for a year or so with volunteer staff, including Alvin Poussaint, the now-renowned Harvard psychiatrist. From civil rights heroes and the people I worked with in the sixties who taught me what "maximum feasible participation of the poor" meant in the War on Poverty, to leaders and government officials who were not afraid to shake things up, I've had exemplary teachers.

For much of this story, I've been a participant-observer—there to record highs and lows, but also involved in the outcome. The people I interviewed for this book were incredibly generous. They made time for me, pulled out their scrapbooks, their old files, even dissertations. They were eager to talk. I wanted most of all to learn what made them stand up in the face of certain danger and persevere despite mind-numbing bureaucracy. "You can take all the setbacks that life has to offer," one of them said, "when the struggle is your life."

Acknowledgments

The first people I want to thank are those who were convinced I should write this book and were there in the beginning to read outlines and early proposals and bug me to get on with the next steps. They include Dorree Lynn, who literally poured her enthusiasm into me and shared ideas, contacts, and all the agonies of trying to publish; Alice Sardell, who will always be the first chronicler of community health centers and was bound and determined that I should follow suit; Ann Zuvekas, who was incredibly generous with her friendship and her great store of knowledge; Karen Davis and Cathy Schoen of the Commonwealth Fund, who supported my research and encouraged my work; and Hank Cole, Jerry Levine, and Cliff Sotnick, who never stopped believing in me.

Then there are the men and women who made health centers what they are today and somehow found time to open the doors to their world, serve as my guides to an ever-growing and always fascinating circle of informants, and review drafts of the manuscript pertinent to their areas: Dan Hawkins, Aaron Shirley, Jim Hunt, Roland Gardner, Barbra Minch, and Paula Gomez.

I interviewed more than seventy people for this book, many of them multiple times. Most but not all are included in the final manuscript; I thank every one of them for their generosity of time and spirit. I also want to thank Susan Rodberg for her unstinting computer support when it really mattered, Jerri Regan for her advice and support and for helping me organize the voluminous material I collected, Jonny Feldesman for help with indexing, and the people who contributed studies and information—especially Michelle Proser of the National Association of Community Health Centers, but also numerous data specialists in state and local health departments and health care organizations.

The book is all the better for the efforts of the staff at Rutgers University Press, especially Audra Wolfe, a terrific and kind editor, and of Sara Rosenbaum, a discerning reviewer.

Two people I miss terribly and think of as midwives to my work are Joanne Lukomnik, whose unquenchable commitment is a model for future heroes of community health, and Marcy Gross, whose great well of spirit survives her.

Finally, my thank-you list must include the originators of the health center model, without whom this story wouldn't have happened. I regret that I wasn't able to interview Count Gibson, who passed away in 2002. I do know that there is a special place in the pantheon for Jack Geiger, who, with all his other contributions, served as a key informant and reviewer of several chapters and was never too busy to stop and mentor a fellow writer. And that pantheon must also include my husband, Bill Culhane, loving, patient, and surely glad the book is finished.

Community Health Centers

Chapter 1

Heroes of Community Health

Community health centers appeared on the national scene in 1965, offering a new way of providing preventive and primary care combined with consumer involvement and cross-sectoral action to address the underlying causes of disease. Most observers gave them little chance of surviving. They were one demonstration program among many, in an era marked by its social experiments.[1] Yet the centers beat back repeated efforts to eliminate their funding, grew to serve nearly fourteen million people,[2] changed the face of care for poor and underserved people, and were selected for further expansion by George W. Bush's White House.[3]

This unlikely story has many heroes: individuals who made their needs known; homegrown leaders who faced down personal threats with courage and dignity; community groups that wouldn't take no for an answer; organizers and young professionals who wanted to help; churches, settlement houses, medical schools, and health care institutions that provided support; and receptive officials who nurtured the early efforts. All of them share the stage with the spirit of the times in which health centers emerged.

The Sixties: Best and Worst of Times

The sixties were not one but several eras. Early in the decade there was a pervasive sense of optimism—as if Camelot dreams in tumultuous Technicolor had burst out of the bland, gray images of the fifties. For many, the changes blowing in the wind were welcome ones. They brought opening and possibility, shared values, wise mentors, and redemptive experience.

Strands of civil rights activism from the previous decade—Rosa Parks, the bus boycott in Montgomery, Alabama, and the involvement of Martin Luther

King Jr. and the Southern Christian Leadership Conference; student lunch counter sit-ins in North Carolina and Tennessee—coalesced and drew national attention. Thousands participated in demonstrations, including the 1963 March on Washington. The assassination of President John F. Kennedy helped spur passage of the Civil Rights Act in 1964, and that same year students headed south to help with voter registration, calling it Freedom Summer. Early the next year people from across the country marched from Selma to Montgomery, where state troopers charged the demonstrators at the Edmund Pettis Bridge, which further raised consciousness and led to the Voting Rights Act of 1965.[4]

By the mid-sixties, civil rights supporters had been joined by protesters against the war in Vietnam. Burgeoning numbers of young people became involved in political activism, driven not just by passion but a personal desire to avoid being drafted to serve in a war they opposed. There was cultural change as well—new freedoms for many; hedonism for some. Youth ruled. "Don't trust anyone over thirty," they cautioned, no longer looking for older mentors. The Freedom Summer of 1964 was replaced by 1967's Summer of Love, when pleasure seekers descended on San Francisco for an endless party.

The drums beat louder and faster. Hopes of political activists faded in the face of prolonged war and more assassinations, first of Malcolm X in 1965 and then King and Robert Kennedy in 1968. Separatism came to the fore, more violent forms of protest. Many retreated into a "politics of lifestyle." Support for group action dwindled as those who were well off expressed their preferences by eating natural foods, buying expensive cookware, and building solar-heated houses in exurbia.[5] Poor people didn't have the luxury of moving to Vermont or Northern California. Stuck with many of the same problems they had before, their expectations raised and then dashed, a small proportion resorted to looting and rioting.

Even as the focus of public attention shifted, the experience of each time lived on among those most involved in one phase or another. No wonder there is a great deal of misunderstanding about those times, and surprisingly little knowledge of what really happened. For example, some critics saw parallels between the profligacy of the culture wars and the government's response to poverty, claiming huge welfare "giveaways" during the sixties.

In fact, Lyndon Johnson's administration (1963–1968) did not propose, nor did Congress pass, any laws to expand cash payments to individuals, widely known as welfare. To the contrary, Congress limited eligibility and instituted work requirements. The welfare rolls did expand—largely because of demographics, increased awareness of existing benefits, and migration from rural to urban areas and southern to northern states with fewer entry barriers. Social spending for elderly Americans of all incomes grew due to indexing of Social Security benefits to labor rates.[6] And health spending grew due to implementation of Medicare to finance care for the elderly and disabled and Medicaid for some of the nation's low-income population. But between 1965 and 1970, when the much-maligned War on Poverty was at its height, funding for the federal Office of Economic Opportunity (OEO), its main attack arm, averaged $1.7 billion annually—less than 1.5 percent of the total federal budget.[7]

Critics also claim that the War on Poverty destroyed family structure and work ethic, expanding the very underclass it was intended to eliminate.[8] Yet the OEO programs initiated in the sixties emphasized jobs and training, economic development and community participation. The people who conceived and ran them opposed the paternalism of welfare. They fought for, and to some degree saw achieved, a caring government with the responsibility to buffer and thus strengthen—not undermine—the free market, end discrimination, and shift the reins of power. Impatient with older methods, they were bureaucrats with little respect for bureaucracy who tried in various ways to involve the people affected. As the early antipoverty workers were fond of saying, "I'm trying to work myself out of a job."

OEO: The Antibureaucracy

Health centers owe their origins to this new concept of government. Early in President Kennedy's administration, many of the nation's leaders had "discovered" poverty, reading Michael Harrington's *The Other America* and holding seminars about ways to improve the lot of the poor.[9] A small group headed by then attorney general Robert Kennedy was looking into the problem of juvenile delinquency.

Richard Boone, who worked with the juvenile delinquency group early on and also helped develop ideas for a domestic version of the Peace Corps, came to the assignment with a background in criminal justice, a healthy disregard for social work professionals and university experts, and a growing commitment to citizen involvement. He remembers one meeting in particular. The attorney general had asked him to bring together a group of local leaders who were attempting to combat poverty. "In addition to these local leaders," Boone recalls, "Kennedy had insisted that the secretaries of labor and what was then Health, Education and Welfare (HEW) be present. There was some uninspiring conversation and then an Indian chief asked to be recognized. He said 'I appreciate being here, but I want to deliver a message. People who say they want to help have been deciding what's good for us for a long time. That's particularly true of the Bureau of Indian Affairs. Please, if something new is to be started, plan with us and not for us.' That registered indelibly in Robert Kennedy's mind, and in mine as well. It was an unusual moment of learning."[10]

Sandy Kravitz, a young social worker with a doctorate in public policy and an interest in public health, became program director for the juvenile delinquency group. He shared the view that existing agencies were mired in the status quo, having written his dissertation on charitable organizations like United Way, and found them unwilling to tackle social change. The group visited such places as Mobilization for Youth on New York's Lower East Side that sought to implement something called "opportunity theory" and were beginning to involve residents of the area. According to Kravitz, Robert Kennedy quickly became convinced that poverty and powerlessness, not personality defects, were the major causes of youth crime—and that what came to be called "community action" was the solution. "He loved the idea, even then," Kravitz says. "We'd go into his office late at night to brief him. He'd put his feet up on his desk and start questioning us. He wanted to know everything."[11]

The attorney general's group was one of several in the federal government that helped persuade President Kennedy to make poverty a major focus of his campaign for reelection. White House special counsel Ted Sorenson asked the Council of Economic Advisors, the Bureau of the Budget, the Justice Department, and other agencies to prepare background papers. The work was in progress when the president was assassinated in November 1963.

On assuming the presidency, Johnson adopted the idea of a campaign against poverty wholeheartedly, establishing a presidential task force and selecting Sargent Shriver, Kennedy's brother-in-law, to head the effort. Boone and Kravitz were part of the team charged with developing a national community action program. Boone continued to advocate for "planning with, not for the people," and the concept was finally translated into the proposal as "maximum feasible participation of the poor."[12]

The legislation drafted by the task force, known as the Economic Opportunity Act, featured community action, a Job Corps to prepare teenagers for the labor market, and the domestic Peace Corps, known as Volunteers in Service to America. The bill was rushed through a Congress keen to memorialize the slain president and signed into law in August 1964. Rather than have existing agencies operate the new programs, OEO—an office reporting directly to the president—was established to run most of them.[13]

Shriver, still splitting time with his old job at the Peace Corps, was appointed as director. Jack Conway, director for industrial unions at the AFL-CIO, was chosen to head up community action. According to his oral history in Michael Gillette's *Launching the War on Poverty*, Conway believed that people should take a break from what they were doing, so he asked Fred Hayes, who had been the development person, to direct operations—in particular, funding of the local community action agencies. Boone had been a police captain, and it might have made sense for him to be in charge of operations, but Conway asked him to take the lead for "the idea side," which included research and demonstrations.[14]

Kravitz, who had day-to-day management responsibility for the research and demonstrations unit, says he asked Conway, "Why me?" and Conway replied, "Because you are the only one with a Ph.D." He was disappointed at first but then realized it made sense. "We had a great deal of flexibility and $65 million to spend—an awful lot in 1964." Boone adds that within community action, the research and demonstrations unit was less visible than operations, drew less political fire, and did not require congressional approval for its experimental efforts.

In another important departure from previous policy, OEO's efforts were designed to avoid city and state governments, whose lack of responsiveness to the poor was seen as part of the problem. Instead, the new programs were administered directly by the federal government, or support was channeled through educational institutions, nonprofit organizations, and community groups, including many that were previously neglected or disenfranchised. Big city mayors and governors, particularly those from the South, resisted this diminution of their political control and patronage and demanded veto power. The compromise—a veto that could be overridden by the federal government— stuck in the craw of state and local officials, and intergovernmental relationships played a major role in subsequent opposition to OEO and its programs.[15]

What ensued was one of the fastest rollouts of a new federal effort on record. The hard-driving Shriver recruited people like himself, often on loan from their "day" jobs. Many staffers came on board before they were processed through regular civil service procedures, going payless for weeks and working fifteen-hour days. They discomfited career civil servants by traveling without authorization and seeking input from nontraditional sources, including activists, protestors, even youth gangs. They played an active role in developing concepts, finding people to implement them, and nurturing the new projects. "We wanted to put as much out there as we could, and then help it survive," according to one participant. This modus operandi was diametrically opposed to the usual government practice—passive review of grant applications, with those seeking funds kept at a distance.[16]

Not only were the OEO staffers the antithesis of bureaucrats, many were short-timers. By the end of 1965, both Conway and Boone had left OEO, but not before the prolific research and demonstrations unit had established that all community action grantees would hire and train citizens from the local area served, and helped launch what became known as "national emphasis" programs, including Foster Grandparents, Legal Services, and Head Start—a new early childhood development effort.[17] Health took a backseat until officials realized that it was an essential ingredient of fighting poverty. In particular, it was clear that the poor children enrolled in the first Head Start projects desperately needed medical care. Not only had many never seen a doctor, one-fourth had serious untreated health problems.[18] The new agency put out some feelers for approaches to providing health services, but staffers were dissatisfied with the responses from HEW and established institutions.[19]

Civil Rights and Health

At the same time, civil rights workers were looking for ways to improve conditions in their own communities and those they had adopted during the struggle for equality. Early on, civil rights meant individual rights—an end to discrimination in schools, housing, voting, and public transportation. It was natural to extend the principles of individual rights to medical schools and hospitals. The battle to integrate these bastions of segregation in the South was a courageous one, aided by the advent of Medicare and federal interest in assuring its implementation in a nondiscriminatory manner.[20] But the organizers also had something broader and more proactive in mind.

Jack Geiger had been active in civil rights since his college days, enlisting in the merchant marine in World War II because it was one of the few nonsegregated services. After several years of juggling demonstrations, graduate studies in physiology, and night work as a journalist, deciding on a career as a researcher and then nearly quitting Western Reserve Medical School, he finally found a way to integrate what seemed to be widely disparate interests. Looking out at Cleveland's grimy skyline, he remembers, "I had a moment of epiphany about the social causes of ill-health. I thought I had invented the field. Of course I learned quickly that the English, French and Germans had gotten there ahead of me."

Still at Western Reserve, Geiger arranged a series of rotations in South Africa with Sidney and Emily Kark, who had developed and implemented a concept known as community-oriented primary care. The Karks had established geographically based health centers in two cities and an impoverished rural tribal reserve called Pholela. Using an epidemiologic approach, everyone in a defined area was considered a patient. The centers collected information about the area's health problems and developed a plan of attack, including health and nutrition services, prevention/promotion efforts, even environmental interventions.[21] Geiger was hooked.

Several years later, in 1964, he was serving as Mississippi field coordinator with the Medical Committee for Human Rights. "That was Freedom Summer, when hundreds of kids came down to work," Geiger explains. "We brought in doctors and nurses to provide medical protection, not just for the white kids from the north but the people in the south laying their lives on the line." It was a dangerous proposition. In June three voter registration workers—James Chaney, Andrew Goodman, and Mickey Schwerner—went missing and later were found murdered under an earthen dam near Philadelphia, Mississippi, the victims of Ku Klux Klan violence.

Among the people Geiger recruited was Count Gibson, chair of the Preventive and Community Medicine Department at Tufts Medical School. Gibson contributed to the effort in many ways, not the least of which was his background and demeanor as a white patrician from Georgia. "Whenever the local police stopped our car," Geiger recalls, "Count would stick his head out the window to speak for the group. His Georgia accent deepened as the summer wore on."

Geiger continues his story: "That fall we kept going back to Mississippi. We had started a small clinic staffed by volunteers and some other efforts to provide local health services. Nothing comprehensive, but the need was staggering. On December 11 we were meeting with a group of leftover civil rights types at the Holiday Inn in Greenville. Everyone was let down and demoralized, fighting over who would get funding from the new OEO Head Start program. Suddenly I remembered Pholela." At that meeting, Geiger described the Karks' model, adding the concept of using health as the entry point for broader social change. "I suggested that a northern medical school, insulated from local political pressures, might be able to start a similar center in Mississippi," he recalls. The room was energized. Flying home together, Geiger and Gibson were grounded in Atlanta and talked into the night. Gibson offered Tufts as the base for a health center, and the two set about to look for funding.

Enter the Health Center Concept

The physician-activists first approached William Kissick in the surgeon general's office at HEW. He referred them to Lee Schorr, who was just about to leave her job at the AFL-CIO for OEO. According to Schorr, Kissick called her and said, "Hey Lee, there's a wild man in my office, and he's got some ideas we can't do much with over here, but I think you people in the War on Poverty would find him pretty interesting." Geiger "materialized" in Schorr's office, and she made an appointment for him with Kravitz, her boss-to-be at the community action research and demonstrations unit.[22]

"On January 25, 1965, I went to see Sandy with my yellow pad full of notes," Geiger recalls. "For two hours I described the health center idea as part of the community action program. But in a classic academic sidestep, we had only requested $30,000 for a feasibility study. Kravitz said no to the $30,000 but offered us $300,000 to start the health center right away." Geiger and Gibson went back to the drawing board, also adding a site at Columbia Point, an isolated and troubled housing project in South Boston where Tufts had been operating a home health program. Geiger says their budget went to $1.3 million in a matter of weeks.

Ideas are translated into government programs in several ways, not the least of which is serendipity—what fills the bill when policy makers are looking for a solution. The community action staffers were "reluctant to use new funds to plug old loopholes," according to Schorr. OEO wanted to avoid "the traditional inaccessible, sporadic and hurried care that was working so badly for the disadvantaged," Schorr says. Neither were they impressed with proposals to change patients' attitudes rather than the system that ill served them.[23]

At the time, most poor people's health care in cities was a matter of riding three or four different bus lines to a charity hospital, only to wait for hours on hard benches for impersonal and episodic services—services that were nevertheless quite expensive. In rural areas, care was often lacking altogether, and in the South the few services available were frequently provided by local physicians who herded minority patients through the back door into segregated waiting rooms.

In contrast, the model Geiger and Gibson were suggesting featured personal health care from teams of physicians and other health professionals, often assigned to follow specific families; convenient locations and a focus on the communities to be served; outreach, child care, and transportation to help the severely deprived patients use the services; attention to the economic and environmental factors that contributed to ill health; and involvement of the patients themselves in how the programs were set up and run.[24]

Thus Schorr and Kravitz were very enthusiastic about the Tufts proposal. But Shriver, who insisted on making all final funding decisions himself, remained to be convinced. Kravitz says the agency head was somewhat suspicious of the concept, feeling more comfortable with ideas he had played a larger role in developing, like Head Start. "And he was not too sure about me. He typically gave me a hard time; liked to call me 'Doctor Strangegrant.'"

"Shriver had his own medical experts review the Tufts proposal," according to Kravitz. "He read us out when he discovered that we had been focusing on the positive comments, kind of like movie publicists picking and choosing among critical reviews. He finally asked Julius Richmond, a physician known for his research on child poverty who was heading Head Start at the time, to recommend a decision." Luckily Richmond was sympathetic to the health center idea, and he saved the day.[25]

On June 11, 1965—six months to the day after Geiger and Gibson had first conceived the idea—OEO approved a grant to Tufts University for one health center at Columbia Point and another at an unspecified site in a southern state. Although organizational work began in the politically controversial Mississippi Delta at the same time, funding at that particular location did not begin for another eighteen months, after much strategizing and a last-ditch sit-in by Geiger and the Tufts medical school dean in Shriver's office.[26]

By then, according to Schorr, the agency had become actively involved in promoting similar health centers and was supporting projects in eight areas, including Denver, Chicago, and the problem-riddled Watts neighborhood of Los Angeles.[27] While individual components of the community-oriented primary care concept can be found in earlier U.S. programs, including turn-of-the-century settlement houses, rural outreach efforts such as the Frontier Nursing Service in eastern Kentucky, some city-operated clinics, and social medicine departments of progressive institutions like New York's Montefiore Hospital, OEO was the first to bring the full-scale model to this country. Kravitz says that Schorr deserves an enormous amount of credit for her leadership: "It would not have happened if not for her dogged persistence." And unlike some of the other "national emphasis" efforts whose management was spun off to other units, the health centers' early growth remained the responsibility of Kravitz, Schorr, and their coworkers.

In June 1966 the still-infant program received a big shot in the arm. Schorr got a phone call from the office of Massachusetts senator Ted Kennedy, who was interested in health services for the people using OEO programs. "Get up there and tell them what they should do," Richmond, still the health center advocate, advised her. Schorr did so, pitching her approach and arranging for the senator to visit the Columbia Point center in his home state. Impressed with what he saw, Kennedy played a personal role in persuading his colleagues that, unlike some other OEO efforts already under political fire, the centers were corruption free, run by professionals, and providing a much-needed service. In April 1967 authorizing language was added to the OEO act, and $51 million was earmarked for health centers. No longer dependent on administrative decisions, the centers had a life of their own. There followed a period of rapid expansion: within a year, thirty-three new centers were funded.[28]

Although Kravitz left OEO in 1966 and Schorr left in 1967, the agency was now committed to the health center program. Boone says that Shriver, originally ambivalent about the centers, "came to hope that they would actually save OEO from what had become the wrath of powerful mayors, leaders in Congress and pessimism in the White House."

The program took on some bureaucratic trappings as administrative responsibility shifted from the research and demonstration unit to an Office of Comprehensive Health Services, still under the aegis of community action. Shriver also established an Office of Health Affairs (OHA), reporting directly to him, to coordinate OEO's health efforts. OHA was first headed by Richmond and then by former Peace Corps medical chief Joseph English. As the Johnson presidency drew to a close, all OEO health programs were consolidated in OHA.

In addition, HEW began to fund its own version of the health center model under a highly flexible demonstration authority. This represented a reversal of previous policy and practice. HEW was peopled with traditional public health types who were uncomfortable with the provision of comprehensive care, favoring "categorical," or disease-specific, education and screening programs run by state and local health departments. A group of what political scientist and health center historian Alice Sardell calls policy entrepreneurs, headed by George Silver, deputy to Assistant Secretary for Health Phil Lee, was able to overcome this opposition.[29]

The early HEW centers were more medical in their approach, but in other respects they resembled the OEO model. Some were nested within neighborhood multiservice organizations, an initiative of the Johnson administration to coordinate efforts of existing agencies. These health centers could look to their parent organizations for some of the nonhealth services, although they were also subject to the internal politics of the sponsoring group. In his master's thesis, Harvard health policy expert David Blumenthal dubbed the effort "Out-OEO-ing OEO." By 1969, HEW had funded twenty-four centers.[30] According to some accounts, HEW planners called for as many as 1,000 health centers serving twenty-five million people to be started over the next five years.[31]

HEW also took steps to refocus its migrant health program, which had been created in 1962 as a response to exposés of farm labor like Edward R. Murrow's "Harvest of Shame." Rather than categorical health department programs that provided little in the way of primary care, or vouchers for local doctors that often ran out before the end of the year, it proposed a comprehensive model with ongoing health and social services involving the patients themselves,

much like the health centers. Bill Hobson, who later returned to head the federal bureau operating the centers, was a young HEW staffer at the time. He remembers the battle over new migrant health regulations, which were strongly
opposed by farm groups and by the health departments that had been running
the programs: "We appealed to HEW Secretary Elliot Richardson, who ruled in
our favor after a marathon hearing that lasted a full day and a half."

Then, Hobson recalls, "it became part of my life goal to enforce the regulations I had fought for." He transferred to HEW's Seattle regional office, where he
developed a plan to substitute comprehensive centers for the categorical health
department programs in the agricultural valleys of the Pacific Northwest, and
visited every valley, organizing migrant worker participation and negotiating the
transfer of authority. In Oregon, Hobson says, there had been one major grant to
the state health department, which took 50 percent for administrative costs and
passed the rest along to counties. "I was on television testifying three times to the
state legislature before we made the switch. The longest holdout was in Hood
River, Oregon, where we were trying to organize a health center for the orchard
workers," he remembers. "Groups backed by the orchard owners who were trying to get control of the grant had our cars followed and threatened us."[32]

The Struggle for Community Autonomy

While health centers were more politically acceptable than many other War
on Poverty programs, there was still opposition from southern governors, organized medicine, and some members of Congress. The need to appease conservatives who supported the Vietnam War was increasingly important to
Lyndon Johnson.[33] And the very nature of the program harbored contradictions
that led to fierce battles between community activists and their sponsoring
institutions.

Early OEO guidance for health centers was quite general. The centers were
to provide a wide range of high-quality ambulatory services in an accessible
"single-door" facility, involve community residents, coordinate closely with
other community resources, and make use of all existing funds, including those
of Medicaid and other health programs.[34] While no preference as to type of
sponsorship was given, and some community action programs and community
development agencies served as grantees, medical schools and teaching hospitals received the majority of grants during the first four years of the program.[35]
These institutions offered political protection, professional credibility, and
experience in administering federal funds.

Even so, as Kravitz puts it, "the themes of maximum feasible participation
of the poor and community empowerment ran through all our efforts. We saw

institutions as unresponsive and we were out to change their culture." One problem was that as time went on, it was hard to find many progressive institutions where people like Geiger and Gibson were strong enough to overcome resistance to meaningful citizen involvement. Those reformers who did challenge prevailing attitudes in medical schools and hospitals were often able to maintain the struggle for just a few years.

Neither were local health departments usually the answer. Of the earliest grantees, OEO found them least successful. Unused to providing medical care and fearful of upsetting private practitioners, they frequently reverted to serving as a conduit for local physicians, as they had in the original migrant health program, without desired changes in the scope, organization, and management of services.

The search for sponsors coincided with confrontations of institutions and, in some cases, OEO itself by community activists, emboldened by years of protest. Early on at the center in Watts, control shifted painfully from the University of Southern California, never comfortable with the level of citizen participation OEO envisioned, to a community organization. The struggle for control repeated itself throughout the country, affecting even the original centers funded through Tufts.[36] Once they had separated from the institutions, many health centers continued to have troubled relationships with hospitals and medical schools over issues of trust and town versus gown cultures. In some areas, the centers found hospitals unresponsive on such questions as staff privileges for their physicians and treatment of uninsured patients referred for specialty or inpatient care.[37]

Out of these conflicts came a reorientation as to health center sponsorship and greater clarity about OEO's expectations. Although there were always some at OEO who persisted in the view that the health care system could be improved by top-down funding to hospitals and mainstream institutions, community organizations, while politically provocative and administratively inexperienced, seemed to offer the greatest likelihood of the structural change that staffers were looking for. The program began to provide training for the centers' administrative staff as well as for the newly empowered board members, and the vague principles of "maximum feasible participation" were finally honed into specific requirements for consumer governance. Guidelines issued in 1970 specified not only job training and a career ladder for neighborhood residents but also two alternate ways to assure consumer input: a center could have either an advisory board, half of whose members were eligible to receive services, or a fully empowered governing board, one-third of whose members were service eligible.[38]

The governance controversies didn't stop growth, and the federal presence had incredible spin-off power. People saw health centers as a model to link health services to jobs, nutrition, and economic development. Grassroots groups heard about the model and adapted it as their own. In Texas and elsewhere, migrant health advocates were able to take advantage of the new HEW support for the comprehensive health center approach. In Boston, organizations from dozens of neighborhoods bereft of health care established centers supported both by federal funds and by city government.

Many of these projects were tilling fertile ground, according to Richard Couto, who has documented earlier activism in southern rural communities that eventually developed health centers. The precedents he studied include the Penn School, established by Quaker abolitionists to assist freed slaves in the South Carolina Low Country, post–Civil War Reconstruction programs, and outposts of the New Deal–era Farm Security Agency, predecessor to today's Farmer's Home Administration.[39] Churches and religious institutions also played a major role in supporting development of the early centers and serving as start-up facilities, just as many of them had sheltered and nurtured participants in the civil rights movement.

The Two Nixons

Health centers' early years were shaped by an unusually creative series of interactions between community activists and receptive officials. But starting with the election of Richard Nixon in 1968, the story shifts to one of political challenge and survival.

Soon after taking office, Nixon announced his "New Federalism" policy, designed to significantly reduce the burgeoning number of programs that had sprung up during the Kennedy and Johnson administrations. Some were to be eliminated, others combined in a few large block grants that would move decision making to the state level. OEO's operating responsibilities were to be transferred to the relevant cabinet agencies, leaving it free to serve as "an incubator for new programs."[40]

At this point Nixon's domestic policies were not as conservative as they would later become. He and many of his appointees believed that government should be actively involved in social issues, but through more traditional means than those espoused by most OEO programs. Thus they supported a massive welfare overhaul with increased financial assistance to low-income families, as well as universal health insurance, with states playing the lead role.[41]

Even as other OEO efforts faltered and funding for the agency itself peaked, health centers continued to benefit from an infusion of new dollars. By 1971 there were 150 health centers in inner-city and isolated rural areas—100 funded by OEO and 50 by HEW.[42] Their survival and growth in an administration pledged to dismantle OEO and discontinue its programs testify to the persistence of the centers' model, strong congressional support, and some unlikely friends in high places.

Nixon appointed a young Illinois congressman, Donald Rumsfeld, to head OEO. Rumsfeld, who also held a White House staff position, supported the continuation of OEO, at least for a while, and fought to maintain the federal right to override a governor's veto over federal funding. He visited health centers and became convinced of their utility.[43] And he used HEW's plans for 800 to 1,000 centers to argue for major expansion, although Nixon eventually chose to expand health maintenance organizations (HMOs) instead, making a mainstream, business-oriented effort the centerpiece of his health services agenda.[44]

As Rumsfeld and his staff began to transfer health centers to HEW, they chose stable organizations with less political opposition. This freed up money to fund some new organizations within the set amount of money available to OEO, but also allowed the agency to keep politically vulnerable grantees (usually in the South) under its protection.[45]

At first, the centers that shifted to HEW found a comfortable home, despite the much larger and more decentralized bureaucracy. But as the transfer neared completion, pressures increased. Nixon's second term was characterized by a turn to the right, more conservative staff, and efforts to force the bureaucracy to conform to his goals. Rumsfeld moved on to other federal positions (and later to his first term as secretary of defense when Gerald Ford replaced Nixon). OEO was reduced to a small vestige of itself called the Community Services Agency, and block grants were enacted for most of its programs, including the local community action organizations.[46]

No longer protected by high-level allies within the administration, health centers faced their first major battle. In 1972 HEW issued regulations asserting that federal support was no longer needed, since the centers could collect reimbursements from Medicare, Medicaid, and private insurers and become self-sufficient. The following year Nixon asked Congress to phase out the legislation under which health centers were funded. House health subcommittee chair Paul Rogers of Florida and Senator Ted Kennedy, now in charge of health for the Senate Labor and Public Welfare Committee, led the fight to fend off both efforts. First, Congress's investigative arm, the General Accounting Office, assessed Nixon's policy and found that dependence on reimbursements was not a practical option for the centers. Medicaid was then and remains today a federal-state program allowing states to set many of the parameters, including payment rates, eligibility, and some covered services. Thus only one-third of the poor were covered across the country. In many states, rates were too low to attract private physicians, let alone cover the broader package of care provided by health centers, and some states refused to pay the centers at all, deeming it a federal responsibility.

Then Kennedy introduced a bill that gave the program its own section in the Public Health Act, delineated required and optional services, and mandated that all centers have a consumer majority governing board—an even stronger commitment to citizen participation than had existed under OEO.

Kennedy remembers the time and attention from members themselves that went into the governance provisions. In a 2002 interview for the Capitol Hill newspaper *Roll Call*, he stated: "We had a markup for three days on the makeup of the boards of the . . . centers, about how many consumers were going to be there and what the power was going to be. . . . And the reason that those . . . health centers have been successful . . . and they're the backbone of service to the poor—is because I think we got it right then."

Although Nixon resigned in the wake of the Watergate scandal in 1974, Gerald Ford, his successor, continued the same policies regarding centers, pocket-vetoing the health center legislation in 1974 and vetoing it outright in 1975. Congress overrode his veto, and the program emerged stronger and better defined than at any time in the past.[47]

As the legislative battle was raging, Ed Martin, a former physician-activist and health center director, assumed leadership of HEW's Bureau of Community Health Services, where the centers were administered. He and his staff took care to adopt the Nixon-Ford rhetoric about self-sufficiency and greatly increased management oversight. They developed and promulgated an index of medical underservice against which applicants' need for services could be measured. They also established an information system, much of which is still in place today, requiring each center to report on numbers and types of staff, patients, and encounters as well as revenues and expenditures. This allowed the calculation of productivity and financial indicators—at first unpopular with the centers, but a major advantage in arguing their case with conservative decision makers.

Perhaps most controversial was the decision to establish many more projects—first in rural areas (and not coincidentally, more congressional districts) and then, toward the end of the decade, in cities. In 1974 there were 158 grantees; in 1980, 872. While the number of grantees now approached early HEW predictions, the new centers tended to be small, and so only about five million people were being served in total—a fraction of the twenty-five million originally projected. Moreover, the centers' stewards implemented a "lean and mean" model, without most of the nonhealth services that characterized the earlier grantees. Since increases in appropriations did not keep pace with the phenomenal growth rate, some of the money for expansion came from cuts in support for the older, more comprehensive centers.[48]

Rebirth under Carter

Jimmy Carter's years in the White House represented a breathing spell for social programs in general and a renaissance of sorts for health centers.[49] Stymied by double-digit inflation, Carter considered but did not propose big initiatives. He asked First Lady Rosalyn Carter to head up a task force on mental health but ended up proposing only a small amount of "glue," or linkage money, for its recommendations. He set HEW to work on a national health insurance plan but failed to introduce legislation to implement it.

Yet Carter did seek significant funding increases for health centers as part of a policy that favored primary care over hospitals and research. Joe Califano, Carter's first HEW secretary, had served as Lyndon Johnson's domestic policy adviser and was sympathetic to at least some War on Poverty programs. A peripatetic activist, Califano took on the tobacco lobby and popularized preventive health, issuing the first in a series of national report cards known as *Healthy People*. He was critical of hospitals' inability to control costs, calling them "obese." His support for health centers, in particular, solidified when he visited the Sunset Park center on the Brooklyn waterfront and discovered his own cousin on the exam table. "We knew Califano's cousin was a registered patient who used our facility," admits Harvey Holzberg, the center's executive director at the time, "and this guy was happy to come in on the day of his visit."

Califano's staff included others who were knowledgeable about the centers. Economist Karen Davis, recruited from the Brookings Institution, had just published *Health and the War on Poverty*, reporting favorably on the centers' potential. Davis's staff included Cathy Schoen, her coauthor on the study, as well as former poverty warriors, policy analysts who had studied health centers, and longtime center director Dan Hawkins from Harlingen, Texas.

From her post as deputy assistant secretary for planning and evaluation, Davis worked closely with those responsible for administering health centers, sometimes questioning the new model for eating into the nonhealth activities that made the early centers unique. She used a network of former colleagues in place at the Departments of Labor and Agriculture to help maintain health centers' cross-sectoral thrust—for example, gaining White House support for an interagency agreement with the Farmers Home Administration to build and renovate facilities for rural centers.

In 1977 Congress, with HEW and White House backing, passed the Rural Health Clinic Services Act, which increased Medicare and Medicaid reimbursement rates and allowed payment for nurse practitioners and physician assistants in rural health centers. The Carter administration also proposed, but did not see enacted, other reimbursement improvements that would have lessened the bind of health centers expected to collect higher Medicare and Medicaid payments.[50]

During discussions about reauthorizing the program in 1978, the health center–hospital conflict resurfaced in the form of proposals by New York senator Jacob Javits and others to fund hospital-based centers without consumer governing boards. Health center organizations objected to undermining the principles of community governance. Senator Kennedy agreed, arguing that "hospitals ought to go the extra mile and meet the governing board requirements" if they wanted health center funding. If some hospitals had seen fit to work with community boards, he said, others could as well. As a compromise, legislation authorizing a small demonstration of hospital-based centers was enacted, but repealed the following year.[51]

On the eve of the 1980 election, health centers were doing well—but they were about to face their biggest challenge yet.

The Reagan Challenge

Early in 1981, the new administration headed by Ronald Reagan hit the ground running. Relying on the advice of ideological conservatives from groups like the Heritage Foundation during the campaign and the transition period after the election, Reaganites had developed a series of policies and a pool of like-minded appointees to carry them out.[52] Almost immediately, the White House proposed consolidation of many additional social programs into block grants to states—this time with none of the hesitance that typified the early Nixon years. Except for Head Start and health centers, most of the original War on Poverty programs were already included in block grants. These were to be simplified, removing reporting and maintenance of effort requirements. The Community Services Administration was eliminated and its programs transferred to Health and Human Services (HHS)—HEW's new name after education had been moved to its own cabinet department in 1978.[53]

The Heritage Foundation distrusted health centers and derided previous expansion plans from the Johnson and Carter administrations, playing on fears that these programs were stalking horses for a nationalized health care system. Reagan asked that a total of sixteen health programs be combined in a prevention block grant and ten programs—including health centers, alcohol and drug abuse, mental health, and maternal and child health—into a block for health services. In addition, funds were to be cut by 25 percent.

Inclusion of health centers in the health services block met with unexpected opposition. Program advocates feared a loss of identity, with good reason: the record showed that without their separate funding streams and special constituencies, blocked programs were less likely to receive funding increases in subsequent years. The centers could also argue that states lacked experience with primary care programs and, left to their own devices, would choose to spend funds instead on services they had been involved with in the past, such as substance abuse, mental health, and maternal and child health. Finally, in some states, competing pressures resulted in low support for poor people's programs generally.[54]

What emerged from negotiations between the GOP-controlled Senate and the Democratic House was a separate block grant for primary care—a block grant in name only. "Subcommittee chair Henry Waxman of California called us in and looked us in the eye," recalls Dan Hawkins, who had left HHS to work for the National Association of Community Health Centers. "He said, 'Here's the deal. There's no way family planning and migrant health can be blocked and still survive state politics. Health centers are strong enough to help save face for the Senate and push through a compromise. I promise we'll write the language together.'"[55] Unlike the administration's proposal, the primary care block grant was voluntary: if states didn't apply to receive it, direct federal funding of health centers continued. States that chose the primary care block had to maintain current funding levels for existing grantees and ensure that they continued to meet all federal requirements.[56]

The administration issued regulations based on its original proposal, trying to ignore the legislative compromise, and the centers went to court. June Green, a federal district judge, refused to enjoin implementation until a state had tried to assume responsibility for the primary care block, and then wanted actual evidence that people would be harmed. Only two states applied. Georgia's application, ruled noncompliant with matching requirements, was withdrawn. HHS approved West Virginia's application in 1983, and the battle was on.

Jacki Leifer, a young attorney who had previously worked for the HHS general counsel, represented the health center association and the West Virginia centers. She remembers the case vividly: "It was one of my first—and still my most important in terms of the program's survival. Several other states were watching closely, ready to file applications if HHS' approval were upheld. Everyone knew it was a pivotal moment."

"The federal officials who had been responsible for health centers' rapid expansion into rural as well as urban America were more or less hostile witnesses for the government, and helped me make my case," Leifer says. "But clearly the star witness was Martha Chapman, the picture of demure West Virginia womanhood in blue-and-white-checked gingham. She wowed the judge by pleading that the block grant would be the death knell for preventive and primary health services to the families who needed them most." The case was decided in favor of the centers. West Virginia, also realizing its residents were losing the benefit of additional money appropriated since the state had taken the block, gave up the fight and handed it back to HHS.[57]

Then Reagan asked again for health centers to be included in a larger, mandatory block grant, but was unable to find a congressional sponsor. Kennedy convinced Utah senator Orrin Hatch, who had originally insisted on carrying the GOP standard, to join him instead in cosponsoring repeal of the primary care block. It took until 1986—two more years of political wrangling—for the repeal to become law over Reagan's veto.[58]

The national health center association played a major role in the congressional events and subsequent legal challenges, having matured greatly since it began in 1971. Tom Van Coverden, a former House Ways and Means Committee staffer, came on to head up a policy analysis shop as the block grant issue was heating up. "I took one look at the job and saw that there was a real threat to the survival of the program," he remembers. "I was brought up on street politics and I relished the challenge." He recruited Hawkins, who had worked with HHS for five years, adding legerdemain with budget numbers to his already considerable knowledge of how the centers operated on the ground. Anticipating the shift of decision making, if not actual administration, to the states, Van Coverden and Hawkins got the Robert Wood Johnson Foundation to support the expansion of health center groups at the state level. By 1986 there were nine regional and forty-two state primary care associations.

The boards of individual centers were also a major source of support. Hundreds of organizations had board member who were movers and shakers in their own communities and could plead their cases personally to elected representatives. Some credit the boards with saving the program. Thus the fight against what advocates called the "block and slash" tactics of the Reagan administration was pursued on local, state, and national levels.[59]

A Time for Resilience

The health center program did take major cuts during the early years of the Reagan administration—the first and only reduction in real as opposed to inflation-adjusted dollars in its history. Appropriations went from $368 million in 1981 to $321 million in 1982—a smaller reduction than the proposed 25 percent cut because Congress added back funds that were earmarked for disease prevention. Instead of instituting across-the-board cuts for all grantees, program officials opted instead to judge each center on the need for its services, efficiency, community support, and whether very small centers had developed sufficient "critical mass" to be viable. Ann Zuvekas, who has studied this period in the centers' history, found that the officials adhered to the standards they adopted. Over a one-year period they reviewed all grantees that had been in existence for two years or more. A total of 187 were phased out, and most others received reduced funding.[60]

After the cutback period, the health center program actually experienced some growth due to increases in regular appropriations and temporary funds to help the centers meeting rising demand due to unemployment. An influx of physicians and other providers from the National Health Service Corps, a program that pays for professional education in exchange for service in an underserved area, drove the expansion and establishment of new sites in urban centers. Some health center directors referred to this inelegantly as the "dump-a-doc" program, as they were asked to absorb new physicians faster than they could add patients and increase revenues. But with these doctors, who were specialty-trained, many more centers could obtain hospital admitting privileges for their staff. The centers also began to network; form alliances; come together in new, more equal partnerships with hospitals; and provide the management of care outside their walls so important to continuity.[61]

The George H. W. Bush administration saw continued action by Congress to increase grant support for health centers, plus another major boost in reimbursement revenues. The Rural Health Clinic Services Act had still left urban centers at the mercy of state Medicaid programs, with payments in some areas as low as $9 per visit. Working primarily with staff of liberal GOP senator John Chafee of Rhode Island, but bringing the Democrats along as well, the health center association helped develop a more comprehensive solution that became known as Federally Qualified Health Centers (FQHCs).

FQHC was enacted for Medicaid in 1989 and Medicare in 1990. The new legislation amended the nation's major health insurance programs for the poor and elderly to include a definition of the health center entity, the package of services to be covered, and the payment method. Health centers and "look-alikes" (organizations that met federal requirements without actually receiving grants) would be eligible for cost-related reimbursement rates, subject to per-visit caps and management screens. For the first time in history, the long-sought integration of the centers with Medicaid and Medicare was possible.[62]

One result was that Medicaid began paying much closer to its full share for covered patients. Another was that it replaced federal grants as the largest source of income for the centers. In 1990 such grants accounted for 41 percent of center revenues; by 1998 the proportion had fallen to 26 percent. During the same period, Medicaid's proportion went from 21 to 34 percent.[63] To some, cost-related payment under FQHC seemed to be bucking the trend to managed care and capitation, but it would survive repeated phase-out attempts. Eventually the FQHC provisions were converted to a prospective payment system that still approximated costs, but in a way that controlled for potential inflation.

Clinton's Record

With the election of Bill Clinton in 1992, the White House reverted to the Democrats after twelve years of Republican rule. The Clinton years offer an important lesson as to why bipartisan popularity and congressional support for health centers have been so essential.[64] The newly elected Democratic administration did not shrink from social causes, proposing expansions of programs like Head Start and AIDS research. But neither did it provide the support health center advocates had hoped for.

During the Clinton health care reform effort, health centers were affected, as were many programs, by White House task force director Ira Magaziner's insistence on forcing everything into the predetermined mold of "managed competition." Nearly all existing health legislation was to be repealed. Scores of programs carefully crafted by Congress over the years, and many state responsibilities as well, were to be rounded up and herded through new private groups known early on as "purchasing cooperatives," or later as "health alliances." A final background paper on health care for the underserved spoke to the rationale for programs like health centers even in the presence of universal coverage, and projected the costs for start-up, development, and nonmedical services unlikely to be covered by the new insurance proposal. Yet the paper presented differing views on whether the programs should be supported through existing authorities or consolidated with insurance funds run by the purchasing cooperatives.[65] This reflected disagreement between those who wanted to "do no harm" to the fragile safety net for the poor and needy and administration representatives who urged the group to "believe in the new system."

During one meeting the president had scheduled to hear the ideas of his task force leaders, he excused himself from the Roosevelt Room to take a phone call from First Lady Hillary Rodham Clinton, who was visiting her terminally ill father. He returned and made a point of saying, "I know there are some good programs out there. Let's make sure we keep them going. Don't reinvent the wheel." Nevertheless it took the intervention of Democratic congressional staff to assure the survival of health centers and other programs.

The battle was repeated when the White House task force was disbanded and HHS took the lead in developing the details of the plan. By then most people realized that the health alliances had no constitutional powers and therefore could not take on regulatory responsibilities. But there were renewed efforts to combine federal health programs, this time channeling the funds through states. To health center advocates, the HHS proposals looked suspiciously like the block grants they had spent years fighting. Again they intervened. The end result, reflected in the Clinton Health Security Act, was to continue separate legislative authorities for programs like health centers, along with additional funds to support development activities. In addition, the centers, as well as other safety net programs, were designated "essential community providers" eligible for special consideration in adapting to the new insurance mechanisms.[66]

Even after health care reform went down in flames, health center program officials within the administration had difficulty getting their requests for budget increases approved. To be fair, there was little discretionary money available—the Reagan tax cuts had seen to that, and Clinton wanted to decrease, not increase, budget deficits. But health centers were rarely in the most highly protected budget category, as were AIDS and family planning. HHS secretary Donna Shalala, who came from and returned to the academic community, expressed a preference for "marrying the health centers to teaching hospitals," rather than expanding the services they provided. Networking proposals advanced by center advocates to better coordinate specialty and inpatient care for their uninsured patients were reinterpreted so it was possible to bypass involvement of the centers themselves. HHS officials also questioned whether health centers were "community friendly," because they were rarely funded through local health departments.

Why didn't the Clintonites see the health center model as fresh and relevant to today's needs? One possible reason was the discomfort of some officials with "poor people's programs." Some believed that any mention of the poor was a political kiss of death. Theda Skocpol, who analyzed reaction to the Clinton health care reform effort in her book *Boomerang: Clinton's Health Security Effort and the Turn against Government in U.S. Politics*, quotes from White House "spin" instructions that cautioned, "We should not even talk about the '37 million uninsured,' because that is not who the proposal is designed to protect."[67] A more humane stance, but still not supportive of health centers, was taken by those who failed to recognize that universal coverage alone would not deal with maldistribution of resources and services. Officials thought they could avoid "two-tier care" by "mainstreaming" the poor. As if to illustrate a major problem with this concept, after the Clinton proposal failed and market reforms proceeded without benefit of regulation, many mainstream plans dropped out of the Medicaid market, effectively precluding participation of poor people.

As had been customary throughout a great deal of the health center program's history, Congress was responsible for most of the funding increases, besting the administration's requests in seven of the eight annual budgets for which Clinton was responsible. Even after the Democrats' disastrous losses in the midterm election of 1994 and the takeover of Congress by Newt Gingrich and his Contract with America, funding held its own and then began to rise again. Between 1995 and 2001, health center appropriations increased 65 percent, from $757 million to $1.2 billion.[68]

A Long, Strange Trip

During the 2000 presidential campaign, Democratic primary candidate Bill Bradley and Republican George W. Bush both embraced the goal of doubling health center capacity, while Democratic nominee Al Gore refused to do so. When Bush took office in 2001, proclaiming the theme of "compassionate conservatism," one item near the top of his list was expansion of the centers.[69] In his first budget message, he proposed to add 1,200 new and expanded sites and increase the number of people served to sixteen million over the next five years, and eventually to double the centers' capacity.[70] Each year thereafter the president continued to push for health center expansion, proposing a second initiative in his 2005 State of the Union address to establish a center in every poor county.[71]

Some detractors saw Bush's support for the centers as an inadequate substitute for the difficult and much more expensive goal of universal insurance coverage. Others pointed out that the aspirational, value-driven, and community-based nature of the program allowed it to bridge the gap between liberals and conservatives. "The Bush health center policy has been quite generous, especially given reduced expectations. Reagan's economic policies limited discretionary spending too, and you didn't see him proposing funds to expand the centers," one observer says.

President Bush's requests for funds to implement health center expansion were generally supported by Congress until 2005, when it more than halved the proposed increase from $219 to $116 million as part of across-the-board cuts in the face of rising deficits.[72] Again in the 2006 appropriation process, federal deficits as well as costs due to Hurricane Katrina squeezed domestic programs— even those in a favored position such as health centers. Health centers received an increase of only $48 million. That was less than 20 percent of the Bush $304 million request, and most of it had already been allocated to preapproved expansions.[73] In addition, depending on how states implemented changes in the Medicaid program, health centers faced reimbursement reductions of $327 million or more.

But even in the paper-thin domestic budget for 2007, Bush proposed a health center increase of $118 million—the largest percentage increase of any HHS discretionary program.[74] Once again he praised the program, citing a report by the Office of Management and Budget that reviewed hundreds of HHS efforts and found the centers one of only ten deserving of the highest effectiveness rating.[75] Despite the setbacks, the reach of the program was actually approaching the early projections most people had called an impossible dream.

"The single most amazing thing . . . is that the health center movement took root at all," according to one policy expert.[76] How have the centers made this long, strange trip when no one would have predicted their survival, let alone growth?

Reasons for Success

Possible reasons for success include health centers' early history as a program that drew less fire than other OEO efforts, the related fact that they were easy to understand and provided concrete services, their bipartisan political support, their ultimate integration with important insurance streams, and their ability to meet or exceed established measures of need, access, and effectiveness.

Design and Early History

Over the years, health centers tended to do well compared with most other OEO efforts. Local community action organizations, the original core of the unit that spun off the centers and their passionate commitment to citizen participation, drew political opposition early. Not only did elected officials feel they were bypassed, according to OEO's Richard Boone, but the local agencies were job-rich, had a flexible mandate, and were viewed as a prize for capture by contending groups of activists. Squeezed between radicals and conservatives, they were subjected to state control in their first year out of the box, and spent most of their life as a block grant. While advocates fought successfully for the survival of community action organizations, funding in real dollars grew only 50 percent from 1970 to 2001.

Head Start, on the other hand, was never block granted and grew a phenomenal twentyfold during the same years—a social experiment adopted into the mainstream, according to OEO chronicler Robert Clark. It filled a niche where there was little competition, helped meet an increasing need for child care, and served as an umbrella for a wide range of activities. Perhaps most important, it is targeted to young children—a group at least some conservatives find difficult to oppose. However, Head Start also has changed significantly since its inception. It channels a significant proportion of funds through local school boards, relinquishing the direct user involvement of the early OEO days, and during the George W. Bush administration has been under pressure to cut "noneducational" activities such as health referrals and parent involvement and to focus almost exclusively on reading preparation.[77]

Health centers experienced less early criticism than community action organizations, defeated multiple attempts at block granting, and saw their funding increase tenfold between 1970 and 2001.[78] As of 2006, their consumer governance requirements—the strongest of any program to emerge from the War on Poverty—remained unchanged. "We grew low and slow, under the radar," Hawkins says, "until we were big enough to make our presence known."

Concrete Services

Some programs that originated with the War on Poverty have been criticized because they offered the elusive goal of economic development without the substance to make it real. Jobs, by and large, did not become available in distressed areas, and people who lived in those areas lacked not only needed skills but also proximity or transportation to firms in the suburbs.[79] Health centers, like Head Start, may have survived because they offered specific, concrete services when and where they were needed. There is also something about health that touches people in a very personal way. "Because of the health care drought in low-income areas, center services were quickly utilized and appreciated . . . easily described and understood," Boone recalls.

Today the centers provide medical, dental, substance abuse, and mental health services; outreach, transportation to care, and social support services; health education; and nutrition, parenting, and child development services. While the nonmedical services of the early days have become narrower in scope and less likely to be paid for directly by federal grants, many centers continue cross-sectoral activities through alternative funding and collaboration with other programs in their communities. Perhaps because of the salience of health, the centers can be used as a base from which to raise awareness of other issues and what might be done about them, create pride, and promote a sense of community, and as an entry point to solving a broader range of problems without raising the same hackles as a more blatantly political program. And by training and employing community residents in career-ladder positions, upgrading infrastructure, and trading with neighborhood firms, health centers actually achieve economic development, albeit on a smaller scale than the earlier community action programs had promised.[80]

Bipartisan Support, Advocacy, and Ownership

Clearly, skilled advocacy and bipartisan support played a role in the centers' survival, along with courageous and committed officials inside the bureaucracy who took an unusual interest in the program and its grantees. Being in the right place at the right time helped. "Civil rights and the War on Poverty were key to the program's birth," according to Dan Hawkins, "and the need to care for the underserved is the key to growth. But the real key to success has always been the community's feeling of ownership over their centers—that's what has sustained and nurtured us through it all." Consumer governance is the health center characteristic that drew the most criticism in the early days and is under fire today from those who would prefer to receive funding without establishing a consumer majority board. At the same time, it has helped assure the program's survival and provided a vehicle for involvement of communities across the political spectrum.

Democratic champions like Ted Kennedy, Paul Rogers, and Henry Waxman have been joined by Republican supporters, including not only moderates like Susan Collins of Maine but also Henry Bonilla of Texas and Kit Bond of Missouri. "Of course many of you know that community health centers are very close to my heart," Bonilla wrote in a weekly column. The centers fill a critical role, he said, because "too often in poor and rural regions of Texas, parents and children are forced to go without proper health care." Bond says that in his state, "I have seen first hand that thousands of children and families have lived healthier, more productive lives due to Missouri's outstanding health centers."[81]

Integration with Public and Private Insurance

Today the integration of health centers with public and private insurance is a fact of life. Importantly, the two approaches—building a service delivery system in areas that lack adequate access to care, and assuring the availability of health insurance—are complementary, not mutually exclusive. Centers still use grant funds to care for all comers in their area without regard to ability to pay, charging the uninsured only nominal fees or a sliding schedule based on income. They also receive insurance payments for those who are covered. Thus while the

mix of patients by payment source for individual centers varies widely, on average 40 percent of health center patients are uninsured, 37 percent are covered by
Medicaid or the State Child Health Insurance Program, 7.5 percent by Medicare,
and 15 percent by private insurance.[82] And although there have been numerous
glitches along the way, most centers have adapted to the demands of managed
care while maintaining their mission—usually by participating in HMOs with
significant Medicaid enrollment or by forming their own health care plans.[83]

Need, Access, and Effectiveness

One indication of the continued need for health centers is the increasing lack of
insurance, due primarily to erosion of employer-based coverage and to growth
in the number of lower income immigrants who do not qualify for Medicaid.
In 2004 forty-five million people—17.8 percent of the nation's nonelderly
population—were uninsured.[84] But even if everyone were insured, people in
many areas would still lack access to health care. The national health center association estimates that thirty-six million people in such areas do not have a
regular primary care provider.[85] In addition, there is more and more evidence
that the sensitivity and responsiveness of health care to minorities matter in
dealing with intractable and in some cases widening racial disparities.[86]

In 2004 over 914 federally funded health center organizations served fourteen million people, including estimated users of newly developed capacity, in
sites as diverse as schools, homeless shelters, migrant camps, and housing projects. The model has spread, so that an additional one million people were
served by similar programs designated as FQHCs for reimbursement purposes
but not receiving federal grant funds.[87] It is likely that a far greater number of
people obtained care from public and private providers who have taken a page
from the health center playbook, although they may lack such center characteristics as consumer governance, nonmedical services, and a firm commitment to
the uninsured.

While they are tailored to meet the needs of individual communities, all
centers must meet federal standards concerning location and service to underserved areas and populations, so designated because of provider shortages,
poverty, and health status problems. Of those served, 91 percent are poor or
near poor, 64 percent are racial or ethnic minorities, and 29 percent were reported as best served in a language other than English. It is an essential part of
the health center mission to assure that care is provided with respect and sensitivity to cultural and linguistic differences. Thus translation and interpreta-
tion are offered according to each area's demographics, with some centers
providing services in over twenty languages.[88]

The centers have been proven effective in numerous statistically controlled studies, answering previous criticism that too few evaluations included comparison groups. Recent research shows that the centers meet or exceed quality measures of other providers—in some cases at lower cost. Satisfaction is high; patients are more likely than similar populations to receive breast and cervical cancer screening and less likely to have low-birth-weight babies or to be hospitalized for a range of conditions that can be controlled with good ambulatory care. And the centers employ a cutting edge approach to chronic disease management and quality improvement that is only now being adopted in the private sector.[89]

Heroes of Community Health

It has been important for health centers to earn their position by meeting and exceeding the standards established by public health experts as well as the competitive marketplace. But my own years in and out of government have convinced me that traditional paradigms are ultimately insufficient to explain the centers' survival and growth against overwhelming odds. A richer palette—one that includes history, political science, and sociology—is more appropriate. And most of all, the personal characteristics of health center leaders have made a major difference between success and failure.

Some of those characteristics are on display in the stories about national figures and bureaucratic champions you have just read. The next five chapters, the heart of the book, will take you to Mississippi, Massachusetts, South Carolina, New York, and Texas. You will meet some remarkable men and women and gain a closer look at their roots in the historic movements for civil rights and social justice, the conditions and culture in their diverse communities, the problems they faced, and their adaptation to changing times.

You will see how the centers they nurtured interacted with widely varying political and economic environments, health care institutions and other safety net programs, levels of insurance coverage, and state/local support. Each center found its own way from near total dependence on federal grants and providers to fully credentialed staff and a sophistication that rivals most large health care organizations with multiple revenue sources. Personal histories focus on different backgrounds and styles, life choices, strategies for overcoming roadblocks, reconciliation and forgiveness—and most of all, how these heroes of community health brought change to their corner of the world.

Chapter 2

Mississippi:

Where It All Began

Driving northwest from Jackson into the Mississippi Delta everything is quiet and green, a lush fertility the only reminder that this place gave birth to an extraordinary period in U.S. history. Explosive and violent, inspiring and redemptive, the civil rights years are still a touchstone of uncommon valor and long overdue change.

The Deep South is no longer America's heart of darkness. Having had to come farther than many northern places on the road to racial justice, in some ways this area is a beacon of hope. But much remains to be done. For one thing, more people continue to sicken and die here than anywhere else in the nation.[1] The struggle for health—indeed, for life itself—goes on.

Rolling hills flatten into fields as far as the eye can see. The town of Greenwood, once the focus of heated civil rights battles, proclaims itself "The Cotton Capital of the World." There are scores of bridges to cross as the Mississippi River tributaries curl in on themselves so many times you can't tell one from the other. It's as though the rivers' push to the sea has been suspended for a time to allow for a more important task—laying down one of the richest and deepest layers of topsoil in the world. In the midst of this incredible natural wealth, there once was hunger.

What It Was Like Before

To hear L. C. Dorsey tell it, the plantation system that survived well into the twentieth century in rural Mississippi meant "poverty, poverty, and more poverty." She grew up in that system, in conditions somewhere between outright slavery and a company town where the boss owned your house, the store where you shopped, and, as the song says, even your soul. People lived in tarpaper shacks, often without wells and privies, let alone running water and sewers. Some families were forced to drink and wash from drainage ditches. The plantation boss sold food on credit, loaded with fat and starches. Rarely were fresh fruit and vegetables available during the fall and winter months. If the boss was kind, he repaired your cabin when the floor fell in. Kind or not, he kept the books, and you never got ahead—never could buy warm clothes, extra groceries, or lumber to fix your own house. Other jobs were out of the question for those who were poor and unschooled.

Unlike other children of sharecropper families who were pressured by the plantation bosses to join in the harvest, Dorsey never missed a day of school to chop or pick cotton. Her father walked her to the bus stop every day, a shotgun on his shoulder. But she tells a heartbreaking story of how, as a precocious twelve-year-old, she carefully measured the cotton her family picked, subtracted their expenses, figured what her father should be paid, and proudly gave him her calculations to take to his next settlement. Expecting him to return with a little cash for the first time, she was crestfallen to learn that the account, as usual, was even. He looked away in shame when she asked what had happened. She knew enough not to make him admit that he hadn't challenged the boss—and to realize that had he done so, the whole family could have been thrown off the plantation.

Home health remedies abounded—some good and others not so good, but none a match for the rickets, scurvy, diarrhea, skin rashes, and injuries that were the result of being trapped on the plantation. Medical care at best was an "account" at a local doctor's office after the boss agreed to a visit. "Most of those doctors made black people use the back door and wait in separate rooms or halls," Dorsey recalls. "And they expected you to tell them what was wrong. They seldom examined you, let alone asked you to undress. Some people later told the health center doctors they had never had a physical examination before."

Imagine being sick and scared, and then to be treated with disdain by the people who were supposed to care for you. And if you were really ill, you went to a charity hospital where, Dorsey says, conditions were so bad her father, diagnosed with terminal disease, hitchhiked nearly 100 miles home to die with his family instead of with indifferent strangers.[2]

Mechanization of the cotton crop had ushered in a new level of suffering. Plantation owners who once had a stake in the health of their field hands had no reason to provide decent living conditions, much less medical care and other amenities (and perhaps couldn't afford to). With no other work to be had in the Delta, thousands of men fled north for industrial jobs, leaving women, children, and old people behind with even scantier resources and services than before. One study showed that between 1960 and 1964, black infant mortality rose 25 percent in the Mississippi Delta, while white infant mortality decreased 33 percent.[3]

Dorsey married at age seventeen, had six children in quick succession, and became a victim of spousal abuse. Somehow she found the courage to get out, joining famed civil rights leader Fannie Lou Hamer in her quest to register voters. She was ready to challenge the plantation owners herself.

"I went to see a bossman known in the Delta for his toughness and asked if he minded if I took his workers to register," she recalls. "He continued to fiddle with his combine all the while I was talking. 'Nope,' he said. Just when I was nearly out of hearing, the boss looked up and added, 'but if you take them, don't ever bring them back here.' In a second, one man could take away another's job, housing, food and pride."

"I never felt so powerless in my life," Dorsey continues. "I tried to think what my heroes would have done. Finally, with a heavy heart, I told the workers I wouldn't take them if they had to risk so much. Later on, they told me they went to register anyway. That was a big lesson for me—first in powerlessness, and in real power. They did it on their own."

Ollye Shirley provides another perspective on Delta life. She grew up outside of Mound Bayou, an all-black Delta town, and attended a one-room school there. "My parents were the teachers," she says. "Their salaries were low, and our supplies were all left over from the white schools. The bus picking up the white kids would pass us on the road, sometimes forcing us into the ditch."

But her father worked part-time in Chicago to provide for the family, and often came home with used books he bought in the stalls there. "He gave us a good start," Shirley says. "In a one-room school the older kids teach the younger ones—a pretty good model. And my parents expected us to go to college, which was rare. Most of the kids dropped out because they had to work the farms. If they finished high school they went north to jobs in the steel or auto industries. It was mostly menial work, but anything looked good compared with a cotton field." When her family shopped in racially mixed Cleveland, Mississippi, she recalls, "We had to sit in the back of the bus, and get off the sidewalk when white people were coming our way. There were times when I was very angry."

In 1949 Ollye Shirley, then fifteen, graduated from high school and enrolled in Tougaloo College, a small, historically black institution in the rural outskirts of Jackson. "It had an integrated faculty, including visiting artists who had retired from Ivy League and Seven Sisters schools in the north. I played basketball, sang in the choir, and majored in English." One outside event made a lasting impression: "The black teachers in the segregated public schools were paid much less than at white schools, and one sued for equal pay. She and her husband were fired, and no one else would hire them."

Things weren't easy for a young black professional. After college, Shirley herself was fired from an interim job while waiting for her first teaching position to be processed. The reason: the principal discovered she had once worked for a man who had challenged the state's doctrine of "separate but equal" after the U.S. Supreme Court *Brown v. Board of Education* school desegregation decision in 1954. That permanent teaching job never materialized. Having met and married Aaron Shirley at Tougaloo, she followed him to Nashville, Tennessee, where he enrolled in Meharry Medical School. There they attended their first civil rights demonstrations ("just a sea of black folks marching, still coming") and began to have integrated social contacts. "I hated to go back to Mississippi," she admits.[4]

Aaron Shirley offers yet another view of the years before the major civil rights breakthroughs. City bred, he grew up in a Jackson, Mississippi, neighborhood where perhaps one-third of the residents owned their own homes. Own or rent, people kept their houses up. His mother, a nurse's aide, was determined that all eight children go to college. "I was eighteen months old when my father died. I never really knew him, but he left three houses to help make our education possible," Aaron Shirley recalls. His older sister became a registered nurse. He himself was one of a few students at his high school selected to take the college entrance exam. Family expectations and a feeling of social responsibility propelled him through Tougaloo and Meharry.

Although he supported civil rights, it wasn't until Aaron Shirley returned to Mississippi in 1960 that he became an activist. He had received a state scholarship for medical school and was obligated to practice in a rural area for five years. He settled on the town of Vicksburg. But from day one, when a white man backed into his car and the police blamed him, called him "boy," he knew there would be trouble. "I was so angry I left my keys in the car and walked home the five miles." By the time he got there, Ollye Shirley had already been warned about the incident by her school principal.

The real challenge came when Aaron Shirley applied to hospitalize his patients at Vicksburg's two major hospitals. "Treating your patients in the hospital is a normal part of what any physician does, but no black doctor had ever had such privileges in Vicksburg," he says. "I was delivering babies in my office. It soon became obvious I couldn't fulfill my obligations without breaking some barriers." He took the issue all the way to the U.S. Justice Department and, in the case of the Catholic hospital, to the bishop. Not until two months before he left, in 1965, was he invited to join the hospital staff.

At the same time, the civil rights movement was taking hold in Mississippi. "When the people working on voter registration asked if I could lend my house and office, I did," Aaron Shirley says. "When civil rights workers were abused, they would come to me. If someone is injured you treat them. As time went on my wife and I became more and more involved." They found that the regular newspaper didn't report incidents against blacks, so they helped start their own paper, with Ollye Shirley as editor. They couldn't get it printed in Mississippi, so they sent it to New Orleans.

There were threats, and more threats. At night they would pile their children into the car, and make house calls armed with a gun. Aaron Shirley took the boys, aged six and nine, out back and taught them to shoot. "I was most afraid of what would happen to my family when I wasn't there," he recalls. "I let it be known that I was not a disciple of nonviolence." The Shirley family moved from a house in a valley, where attackers could shoot down on them, to one on a hill.[5]

The Will to Overcome

L. C. Dorsey, Ollye Shirley, and Aaron Shirley came from different backgrounds. What they shared was the deep humiliation of being treated as less than human, and the will to overcome—for themselves and others. They all earned doctoral degrees and more than repaid the chances they were given.

Aaron Shirley made a difficult decision to stay in Mississippi. He explains that he applied and was accepted as a pediatric resident at the University of Mississippi Medical Center—part of the ultratraditional institution known as "Ole Miss." The first black person ever to do so, you might call him the Jackie Robinson of Mississippi medicine. "I had five years of experience, and I was there to be a doctor—just doing what came naturally. I had no idea I was such a symbol. Later I learned that the black nursing assistants would come up to my floor and watch me," he says.

For ten years, Aaron Shirley says, he was the only black pediatrician in the state. He has since made it his business to help nearly 200 black men and women become health professionals—challenging admission policies, combing Mississippi for applicants when the schools said there were none, raising questions about those who were rejected. Most of them remain in the state today.

Ollye Shirley pursued a career in teaching and child development, earning a doctorate in education along the way. She worked for the group that brought the Children's Television Workshop, sponsor of *Sesame Street*, to Mississippi, and served as president of the Jackson School Board, where, she recalls, she had a chance to right some wrongs. She fired the man who caused her to lose her first teaching job, and gave a plaque to the teacher who couldn't find work because she had pursued equal pay. "That woman had been punished for fifty years," Ollye Shirley says. She also developed a new relationship with the young man who drove the white school bus and terrorized the black kids outside of Mound Bayou. Later he became a schoolbook salesman, seeking and receiving her help with his business and Aaron Shirley's advice with his medical problems.

Dorsey had perhaps the longest journey. While working with voter registration, she heard about the new health center that was being organized in the Delta and applied to work there. Soon she passed the high school equivalency exam given by the center's education program and was put in charge of training community health workers. She became deputy director and then director of the farm co-op the center organized.

Dorsey says she took advantage of college classes offered at the center through a local college and under the tutelage of senior staff who had faculty appointments at Tufts Medical School. When she left the center, she was admitted directly to a masters' program in social work at the State University of New York (SUNY) at Stony Brook. That was rare even in those days, when some schools gave academic credit for "life experience." Dorsey graduated with honors, returned to Mississippi, put all her children through college, and then worked nights at a nursing home in Washington, D.C., while earning a doctorate at Howard University. The next time she came back to Mississippi, it was to run the health center where she got her start.

Asked when things finally began to get better, Dorsey replies: "When I got my first pay check from the health center. It was free and clear, not like any plantation pay." Then, on reflection, she adds: "I really knew it was better when I saw what the health center did for people. There was money for transportation and prescriptions, even evening hours for people who worked in the fields. It made for an ease and peace we hadn't had before. And the doctors weren't like those we were used to. You felt clean and cared for. They touched you."

What made these three exceptional people, and others like them, stand up against such dangerous and overwhelming odds? Among others, Aaron Shirley remembers that Fannie Lou Hamer used to say she was "sick and tired of being sick and tired." "Maybe it was personality, maybe the way we were reared," says Ollye Shirley. "Some people are in hopeless situations and can't find the resources. We figured out how to do it." It also helped to have educated parents, she says, but her grandparents didn't go past the third grade, and they supported civil rights. "They didn't take any crap. And because of them I knew losing my job was nothing compared to the torture, beating and killing that others had endured."

A Health Center in the Delta

As people like L. C. Dorsey and the Shirleys were coming into their own and the civil rights movement had begun to make inroads into the pain and hopelessness of southern black life, Mississippi saw the establishment of two precedent-shattering health centers. In some ways it's the flip side of the national events described in chapter 1.

The Tufts-Delta Health Center in Mound Bayou, Bolivar County, came first. While Jack Geiger and Count Gibson were traveling back and forth from Boston to Mississippi, and hundreds of other civil rights workers were adopting the state as their own, native Mississippians were pushing for a solution to the terrible health conditions they had been struggling with over the years. Among them was Robert Smith, a black physician and activist who had been involved in civil rights since his days at Tougaloo College, completed medical training at Howard University, and returned to Mississippi to practice.

Smith recalls having been at a dinner party with Medgar Evers, head of the local National Association for the Advancement of Colored People (NAACP), one night in June 1963. As Evers was returning home from that dinner, he was shot down in his own driveway. "I remember my despair, and anger. This place was sweltering in anger," Smith says. "The week after Medgar was killed, I stepped in deeper." Mike Holloman and Walter Lear of the black National Medical Association were asking for help in dealing with the American Medical Association (AMA). Because the AMA tacitly allowed segregated medical societies at the state and local levels, hospitals that required their physicians to be AMA members could exclude black doctors or have a "colored" division. Smith went to picket the AMA convention in Atlantic City, New Jersey—an event that drew national media attention. Later he was fired from his job at a state hospital, and for some time thereafter he focused on doctoring poor blacks without health care and civil rights workers whom other physicians refused to treat.

"There were only twenty-five to thirty black physicians in private practice to serve 800,000 black Mississippians. A lot of them had succumbed to the hostile environment and left the state," Smith recalls. There were safety net providers in some areas, organized around small, poorly equipped black facilities such as the Knights and Daughters of Tabor and Sarah Brown hospitals in Mound Bayou. People paid twenty-five cents every three months to see a doctor if they became ill. Other blacks were relegated to segregated and poorly staffed wards and out-patient departments at some general hospitals. "Mississippi was like a Third World country," Smith says. He remembers that 30 to 40 percent of the children had intestinal parasites, and when people did get care they showed up with un-treated hypertension, diabetes, and heart disease.[6]

In 1960 black infant mortality in the state was 54.4 deaths per 1,000 live births, more than twice the rate for whites and 25 percent higher than black infant mortality in the nation. In some counties, particularly in the poverty-stricken Mississippi Delta, black infant mortality rates were greater than 60 per 1,000 live births.[7] The reasons went far beyond lack of medical care. That year the U.S. Census reported that two-thirds of all housing for blacks was substan-dard. In rural areas, 75 percent of the homes had no piped water, and 90 per-cent had no toilets, baths, or showers.[8]

In 1964 the Medical Committee for Human Rights (MCHR) took on the job of caring for those who had come to work in Mississippi's Freedom Summer project, with Smith serving as volunteer southern coordinator and local contact. Health professionals from many backgrounds and specialties throughout the na-tion participated. "It was like a quilt of the country—a brilliant, innovative and diverse group," Smith remembers. They couldn't help but be engaged by the on-going health problems of local blacks. But most of them didn't stay. Two who did were Geiger and Gibson. "They developed a love affair with Mississippi, using every opportunity to come back," Smith says. "We met frequently." After the summer Smith, serving as the sole state-licensed practitioner at the isolated volunteer clinic MCHR had established, argued strongly for a more permanent answer.

Thus the idea of a health center that embraced multiple resources—legal, environmental, social, and medical—came not only from Geiger's experience in South Africa but more directly from the civil rights movement in Mississippi. As described in chapter 1, Geiger and Gibson sold the new concept to the Of-fice of Economic Opportunity (OEO), the War on Poverty's action arm in Wash-ington, D.C., and in June 1965 a grant was forthcoming for centers in Boston and "a rural site in a southern state."

While the location was vague to placate OEO director Sargent Shriver and get around political opposition, the concept had been developed with Missis-sippi in mind. But where? Geiger says he and Gibson considered various places, rejecting some they thought unsafe for an integrated staff, some because no building was available.

Here the story shifts back to Tufts and the role played by John Hatch, a black southerner who met Geiger and Gibson while he was serving as director of community relations for the Boston Housing Authority. What Hatch really wanted, Geiger recalls, was to be involved with the health center planned for the South. He was welcomed with open arms. "Late in 1965, John set off for Mississippi to scout sites. We didn't hear from him for weeks. Given the risks, we were scared to death." Finally Hatch checked in. "He'd been picking cotton around the state—the best way to find out what was really going on."

Geiger says it was Hatch who recommended the mostly black town of Mound Bayou in Bolivar County. It had a black hospital in desperate need of financial and professional support and a black power structure interested in a health center. What's more, the surrounding area offered good potential for community involvement. Geiger agreed but pursued a diversionary strategy, letting it leak that Tufts had settled on an integrated town where the white physicians, the state medical society, and the health commissioner were strongly opposed to a federal program. Then he and Gibson met with the AMA and appeared to "settle" for Mound Bayou—their first choice all along. Even then, despite substantial covert support, local physicians wouldn't go on record in favor of the center.

In retrospect, Geiger says, it may have been fortunate that it took until early in 1967 for Shriver to sign off on the site. The long delay allowed time to organize in Bolivar County from the grass roots up, rather than having existing leaders assume management of the center. "That was John's real contribution. He's the best community organizer I've ever known." Hatch worked with hundreds of local people to develop ten health associations; they in turn formed the North Bolivar County Health Council, which became the center's advisory committee and, ultimately, its governing board. The council was chartered not just for health care but as a community development corporation, covering a wide range of activities. "We also trained local residents as medical secretaries, typists, and community health workers," Geiger recalls. "By this time we were living in trailers near the center site. One morning I got up to find fifteen people on my doorstep. They had heard about a job opening and waited all night to apply. The demand for work was so great we decided that the health associations would nominate candidates for the jobs we had." One of those hired was L. C. Dorsey.

The health center opened its doors in a small church parsonage, using the living room for waiting, the bedroom for exams, and the kitchen as a lab. People from the community "sent scouts," Geiger says. "First ten people came, then twenty, then eighty. The numbers grew every day."[9] Early in 1969 the *Wall Street Journal* profiled the center, by then in a modern, 4,000-square-foot facility, and reported that 5,000 of the area's 11,000 residents had been treated.[10]

To oversee the center's bustling maternal and child health practice, Geiger recruited Helen Barnes, a native Mississippian. Barnes had attended Hunter College in New York City and medical school at Howard University, worked for four years as a general practitioner in Greenwood, Mississippi, to pay off a state scholarship, and then trained in obstetrics and gynecology at Kings County Hospital in Brooklyn. "Jack spoke with me," she remembers. "I interviewed at Tufts and visited the center site. It was still a hole in the ground. I said I'd come back when the hole was filled."

Barnes's Brooklyn colleagues didn't think much of her decision. They warned her that her education wouldn't be appreciated, that she wouldn't be treated with respect. But Barnes knew what she was facing. "I had paid my first poll tax when I moved to Greenwood in 1960," she recalls. "It was a scary time. The Citizens' Council threatened to have a white man fired from his job if we didn't end our doctor-patient relationship. Black doctors weren't supposed to treat white patients." And on a personal level, she had to back off a friendship she had developed with a white woman. On the other hand, the police chief was supportive and offered to introduce her around when she first came to town. "You work with what you've got and change it," Barnes says. "The need was great in Mississippi, and I always knew I'd come back."

Her approach to medicine went far beyond the standard government formula for maternal and infant care. But it wasn't until Barnes started working at the center that she understood just how social science, environment, and medical care all came together. "If mothers and babies don't eat, all the medicine in the world won't work. We called Washington and said 'Look fellows, we've got to be able to write prescriptions for baby formula,'" Barnes recalls. Two nurse midwives, Sister Mary Stella, a Sister of Charity from Indiana, and Elsa Johansen from Sweden, provided the prenatal care. "They and two ladies they trained from the community would be out all day with a bag lunch, making house calls and showing new mothers how to care for their newborns. They'd come back to the center and tell us where home repairs, window screens, wells, and privies were needed," Barnes says. "For deliveries, we needed hospital space and standards. We took over an abandoned emergency room at the hospital, cleaned, stripped and painted the walls, scrubbed the floors, and installed screens."[11]

Her can-do attitude was typical of other center activities as well. Home improvements and sanitation were an integral part of the agenda. Geiger, now serving as executive director, became infamous in rigid government circles for prescribing not only baby formula but all kinds of groceries. After all, he says with a smile, "the last time I looked at a medical text, the specific remedy for malnutrition was food." The center's farm co-op, a more permanent response to the problem, was born not only of hunger but also from the realization that growing crops was one thing the Bolivar County residents could do well. Using the area's black churches as a base, Hatch recruited nearly 6,000 people as workers/owners.

"The people of Bolivar County were unemployed and hungry in the midst of the country's richest agricultural area," Hatch explains. "But they wanted jobs, not relief." In addition to the farm co-op, the center started a child development program, a bookstore, an education department, and a career-training program. In the center's first decade, Geiger recalls, its high school equivalency and professional preparatory programs established links with colleges, mentored candidates, and "helped to produce five physicians, seven Ph.D.s, two environmental engineers, more than a dozen RNs, a half dozen social workers, a score of LPNs and the first ten registered black sanitarians in Mississippi's history. All this from the third poorest county in the United States."[12]

The center recruited Andy James, a sanitary engineer from Ohio, to launch a major environmental improvement program, digging wells and sanitary privies and controlling rats, insects, and other carriers of disease. "Some of the red hand pumps from the wells we dug can still be seen in Bolivar County," according to Geiger. There was also a portable acute-care package—hospital bed, chemical commode, generator—that made it possible for seriously ill patients to be cared for at home. Organizers of other early health centers funded by OEO, including those in Lee County, Arkansas, and the South Carolina Low Country, visited the Tufts-Delta center and modeled their efforts after its sanitation, home health, and other innovative programs.

Goin' to Jackson

Meanwhile, a group of black Mississippi physicians had targeted Jackson and its surrounding counties as another health center site. They included Aaron Shirley, Robert Smith, and Shirley's practice partner, James (Andy) Anderson. Anderson had grown up with Shirley and gone to Morehouse College in Atlanta on the recommendation of Shirley's sister. Like Shirley, Anderson graduated from Meharry Medical School. Then he started a practice in McComb. "I got in a lot of trouble," he chuckles. That was where he had first met Bob Moses, a renowned civil rights leader. "Bob was standing on the corner teaching people how to vote. People who didn't like what he was doing came and beat him up. I was his doctor, and we got to be good friends. Two years later, we all got together in Jackson, started talking about health care."[13]

During his residency at the University of Mississippi Medical Center, Shirley had seen the sickest babies from all over the state—and the roots of their problems in malnutrition and lack of prenatal care. Caring for newborns at St. Dominic's Hospital, the school's affiliate, he recalls, white mothers always accepted him, but he was the primary caregiver for black babies. "By then the floors of the hospital were no longer segregated, but the rooms were. Every black mother and baby I had were put in the same two rooms. I always knew where to go." Shirley remembers the time Anderson had delivered a premature white baby, weighing two and a half pounds: "The nurses were upset. It was the first time a black physician had delivered the baby of a white woman at this hospital. I'm convinced they didn't care if it survived." But, he says proudly, "that baby has now finished graduate school."

Shirley finished his training in 1967, using his "spare" time helping to document hunger in Mississippi and bringing Senator Robert Kennedy to witness the conditions that so influenced his brief run for the presidency the following year. Then Shirley started a private practice with Anderson in Jackson. Having met Geiger and learned of the health center in Mound Bayou, he also helped out there two days a week. "I'd drive up and back the same day, get to my office around 8 P.M. and work until midnight," he says. "One night Andy and I were sitting there and a woman brought in a baby, stiff and dead. We called the coroner. At the inquest we learned that she had been to the emergency room, where they gave the baby a shot and a prescription. She didn't have the money to fill it. She just sat there and cried. After the baby died she'd been trying to warm it with a heated iron wrapped in a towel."

Shirley and Anderson knew they had to do something. Too many of their patients couldn't pay. And even with free medical care, there were no resources for prescription drugs and other services. "We asked Jack Geiger to help us put together an application for a center here, and he did." By this time, OEO was flush with money for health services, and eager to support projects in Mississippi. But the political barriers were even greater than in Mound Bayou. A federal health center aimed at the black population in the state's capital and largest city drew widespread attention and opposition from the medical society and the health department. Alton Cobb, a former state health officer, said later: "We were defensive. Our attitude was that the program was mainly for black people, and we wanted to say they were already well off and didn't need any assistance. . . . Things have come such a long way since then."[14]

Then, too, the new center lacked the "cover" of a major university. "Educational institutions were exempt from being vetoed by the governor, and Mound Bayou's grantee was Tufts. We were a homegrown group subject to the governor's approval," Shirley explains. That was problematic because "blacks would choose and hire the staff, at the same time as we were trying to participate in the political process. We wouldn't have to bow and scrape any more." Governor John Bell Williams vetoed the grant. One reason given was that Shirley's salary as executive director—$30,000 a year—was too high. The proposed health center became the topic of hearings by congressional committees and the American Public Health Association.

Shirley's involvement with a thorny local issue seemed to complicate things, but ended up winning some important allies. State highway patrol and city police shot and killed two students at Mississippi's Jackson State College in May 1970. Shirley was checking at the morgue, trying to locate a missing student, and working with Charles Evers, Medgar's brother, to prevent more violence. Anger was running high, not least because the Jackson shootings followed those of four students by National Guard troops at Kent State University in Ohio just a few days earlier. "The governor issued a statement that I was using Jackson State to intimidate the feds into overriding his veto of the health center—accusing me personally of threatening to incite riots," Shirley says.

He was treated very differently by federal officials. "I got a phone call from Don Rumsfeld, head of OEO and also an adviser to President Nixon," he continues. "Rumsfeld wanted to meet with the parents of the kids who had been shot. I helped arrange that. Afterwards I took him and his aide to the Tropicana, a restaurant in the black section of town. We had pork chops, black-eyed peas and corn bread," Shirley recalls. "It was important that I was born and raised and trained here. I was able to set the record straight. I wasn't imported. I was one of us who had equipped myself to stand the test. They couldn't question my legitimacy." Ten days later, the governor's veto of funds for the health center was overridden.

On the wall above Shirley's desk today is the framed brown wrapping from that first application, saved and sent him by their OEO project officer. The return address is his old private practice. When the Jackson-Hinds health center opened its doors, Shirley's and Anderson's patients were the first to enroll.

Anderson picks up the story. "We started in the Sunday school room of my church, Cade Chapel Baptist, in Jackson. Aaron was the executive director and I was the medical director, but we both always saw patients." He points to a photo of an old bus. "We bought a bus up in the Delta and took a trip to Philadelphia, Mississippi, to see a Head Start center. The bus didn't make it back. But when we opened a site in Utica, in rural Hinds County, we hauled that bus down here. We used the front for waiting and the back to see patients. Our dentist would take a steel chair, and on a good day he'd set it up outside." The bus was followed by a modular facility on property the center bought from a white landowner who wouldn't back down when his store was shot up and his wholesalers threatened. He took the risk out of concern for the poor blacks in the area. "I saw their teeth wore down to the gums," the man later told a local paper. "They didn't have any health care. . . . It's a terrible thing to need medical attention and not be able to get it, no matter what color you are."[15]

Like the center in Mound Bayou, the Jackson-Hinds center focused not only on medical care but on other barriers to health as well. "Children with chronic diarrhea received a medical assessment, and then we checked their water supply. If they had parasites, we checked their sanitary facilities. If they were malnourished, we got them food. We stretched the definition of primary care to privies and wells," Shirley says. "We developed respect for the things that caused people to be sick," Anderson explains. "If someone is beaten, you treat him. If he's hungry, you feed him." That broad definition of health was at the core of the governor's next challenge.

Just months after the center's opening, Governor Williams went to state court to freeze its funds. Unhappy with the fact that his veto had been overridden, he claimed the health center's activities exceeded those described in its corporate charter. OEO director Rumsfeld sent Justice Department lawyers to help develop a new charter with broader definitions, like the community development corporation in Mound Bayou. The community board running the health center had the same members, but now it was known as the Mississippi Civic Improvement Association. Attorney General John Mitchell, later of Watergate fame, filed suit in federal court to prevent the state's interference with a federal program.[16] The center reopened and kept going, but Shirley recalls that it had to fight a governor's veto each of its first three years—twice under Williams and the third under Bill Waller, who had a reputation as a liberal but was "just smoother than his predecessor."

They weren't alone in their efforts. "We hired Bennie Thompson, now a U.S. congressman, as a social worker and community organizer when no one else would give him a job," Shirley says. "We helped all our adult patients register to vote. Our survival depended on massive community support."

A Long Time Coming

"It was ten years after the bus rides, voter registration drives, and Medgar Evers's death before things began to change," Helen Barnes says. "You have to appreciate that these were Medgar's children. They went to jail in a minute if they thought it would help." And besides the need for legal and political action, there were issues regarding the quality of life. Barnes had expected to spend four or five years in Mound Bayou and return to New York. Instead, she stayed in the state but moved on to the University of Mississippi Medical

Center in Jackson after only two. Despite friends and allies and monthly care packages from Brooklyn, the culture shock got to her. Rural Mississippi in the sixties was a lonely place to be. "There was nowhere in 200 miles to go to a movie or a zoo. Clarksdale, the nearest large town, was just a big Mound Bayou."

When change did come, it was largely through electoral politics. Six of John Hatch's community organizers became mayors of Bolivar County towns with majority black—but previously disenfranchised—populations. That began the long process of providing decent roads, running water, sewers, schools, and housing to those who lacked them.[17]

The power of the ballot box made itself felt in Jackson, too, and around the state. In 1971, with the help of a few outspoken whites, 3,500 black Democrats held their own convention at Jackson State College and nominated Charles Evers, then the mayor of Fayette, for governor. The first seconding speech was given by Fannie Lou Hamer. Only it wasn't a speech, but a gospel song: "Precious Lord, Take My Hand." The song became a duet with Evers, and then the whole auditorium was rocking.[18]

Evers's nomination was largely symbolic, as registration and voting were still problematic for blacks in many areas where whites controlled the process. But blacks and their supporters, known as the Mississippi Freedom Democratic Party, elected a substantial number of delegates to the Democratic National Convention the following year. When some of the blacks were seated, whites in the Mississippi delegation walked out, leaving the Freedom Democrats as the state's official delegation. A decade later, even intransigent white politicians were seeking black support.

The health centers saw changes, too. The 1973 transfer of their funding from OEO to the Department of Health, Education and Welfare (HEW) meant that Jackson-Hinds was funded under different legislative authority and therefore no longer subject to a governor's veto. But at HEW, most administrative decisions were made by ten regional offices, often staffed by older white men who were not sympathetic to community-based programs run by black people. "They were state-oriented types who looked for ways to make it miserable for us," Shirley says. One example: the center moved to a new building approved and funded by OEO before the transfer, but the HEW regional office in Atlanta, which now had jurisdiction, refused for months the funds to pave the new facility's parking lot.

Things were more complicated for the flagship center in Mound Bayou. In 1971 Geiger decided to take a position as chair of community medicine for a new medical school just starting at SUNY Stony Brook. Count Gibson had already left Tufts for Stanford two years earlier. The center's board requested and OEO agreed that SUNY Stony Brook would become the grantee. But according to Geiger, the following year the black mayor of Mound Bayou, along with some powerful political allies, convinced OEO to turn the center over to the town officials. This was one case where having the black power structure involved didn't work to the community's interest, Geiger says. "OEO didn't understand that the town was quite small and predominantly middle-class, while most of the center's patients and governing board members were drawn from the much larger numbers of rural poor in the surrounding area," he explains. The town leaders had tried before, unsuccessfully, to gain control of the center. That effort had resulted in a separate grant from OEO to keep the local hospital alive. Now the two grants were combined, and the inefficiently operating hospital was draining the health center's funds. Geiger also recalls that leadership positions were filled with relatives of the mayor and other town officials. "For some ten years, they ran it into the ground," he says.

Jackson-Hinds, on the other hand, prospered despite hostility from the regional office. It didn't face the same local infighting as Mound Bayou and instead became the "go-to" organization when other communities, like Canton, Meridian, Laurel, and Vicksburg, needed help with developing and operating health centers. The center started its own precedent-setting programs, including mental health services, housing for the elderly, and even school-based projects to prevent teen pregnancy and deal with its consequences. High school students received counseling, tutoring, and health care—including contraception. While many towns more liberal than Jackson have succeeded in blocking such services, the Jackson-Hinds center slowly won the trust of teachers and parents by providing physicals for the sports teams, then expanding to other activities.

By 1979 Jackson-Hinds had become a national showplace. That year, a group of federal bureaucrats from a committee studying child health toured the communities served by the center. Traipsing around in a muddy yard outside a tarpaper shack, the visitors saw the barrels of water the health center workers had delivered, and the window screens they had installed. An invitation to come inside was forthcoming only because Shirley knew the people by name, and they knew and respected him. A small child lay in his crib, much too quiet and withdrawn compared with others his age. That evening, the group learned of plans for an intensive child development program, which would provide hours of stimulation and bonding every day. The mother and child in the tarpaper shack would be the first to enroll.[19]

Then the center at Mound Bayou began a comeback from its years of eclipse. In the early eighties, federal authorities demanded that a new governing board be formed and that the primary care facility, now known as the Delta Health Center, sever its relationship with the hospital.[20] L. C. Dorsey returned as executive director in 1987, serving until 1995. According to Geiger, "She did a marvelous job, despite threats on her life from 'unknown individuals.' They did not go quietly into the night." Under Dorsey's direction, the center, which had built a new facility, established major satellites in Washington and Sunflower counties. It also began to provide home health services in Washington and Coahoma counties, developed a wide range of specialty care, and diversified its revenue sources. "When I took over most of our money was from federal grants," Dorsey says. "By the time I left 75 percent came from Medicaid, Medicare, other insurance and private pay patients."

No Free Lunch

As was true elsewhere in the nation, the Mississippi centers' record of achievement was not without costs. The focus on a leaner medical model meant that the core federal grant no longer paid for digging wells, building privies, developing farm co-ops, and offering a host of other "nonhealth" activities. Because of improved economic and political conditions, the health centers no longer had to provide sanitation and water services themselves, or the same level of job training and employment. But the dispersion of responsibility to multiple groups with widely varying priorities did make a coordinated, community-wide assault on the root causes of ill health that much more difficult. For the nonhealth and social support services that are still needed, center directors have had to become even more entrepreneurial than before, seeking alternative means of support. Some were better at it than others, and Shirley claims that the centers that don't find a way of continuing to do these things simply lack the will.

Adding to the pressure was the need to collect payments from Medicaid and other third-party payers and adapt to the demands of a competitive marketplace. Even where competition for the poorer and sicker population they served wasn't an issue, the centers were expected to behave as if it were. That translated into less time for doctors to spend with patients, more stress, and at times a negative impact on quality of care.

In Jackson, moving into the modern age meant networking with other providers and preparing for involvement in managed care. In 1993 Shirley, always the visionary, was one of twenty-some Americans from a wide range of professions to be awarded a no-strings MacArthur Foundation "genius" grant of $350,000. He applied the funds, and most of his efforts for the next several years, to his dream of renovating a huge bankrupt shopping mall into a modern medical facility, bringing economic development and a broad array of health services to one of Jackson's neediest areas. But he was dealing with institutions the health center folks hadn't much trusted over the years. Ann Zuvekas, who has written about this period of Jackson-Hinds's history, observes that when financial setbacks at the health center gave Ole Miss a controlling interest in the mall venture, failure to bring the center's remaining staff and board members along exacerbated their distrust. They withdrew from negotiations, causing Shirley to leave his beloved center and his old friend Anderson.[21]

The upshot: the gleaming Jackson Medical Mall is indeed a testament to collaboration and a successful showplace that attracts visitors from throughout the country. The mall foundation that Shirley heads receives several federal networking grants and provides some of the health education and school-based services Jackson-Hinds was forced to relinquish because of its budget problems. The University Medical Center has moved its outpatient clinics to the mall, where its specialty services are a resource for all of the state's citizens, and the state health department leases space for several of its health promotion programs as well. But it didn't work out for Jackson-Hinds to occupy the primary care suite, as originally planned. Instead, Aaron and Ollye Shirley's son, Terence, an experienced center director, manages the mall's primary care services. Jackson-Hinds presides over its own new state-of-the-art building several miles away and operates a total of five sites, three of them in surrounding rural areas.[22]

It wouldn't be the last time there were problems between a far-sighted health center entrepreneur, networking with the power structure and other health care providers, and center staff who remain concerned with day-to-day services. And it wouldn't be the only time a group that had fought for independence from hospitals and state government had trouble participating in a more equal partnership with those same institutions.

Your Brother's Keeper

Now the pockets of rural poverty in Mississippi are fewer, yet the problems seem more intractable—unemployment, drug abuse, alcoholism, depression. Blacks, who once fled the South in great numbers, are returning to the region.[23] But urban or rural, the influence of extended family is less prevalent, and the drive for education and upward mobility has passed many by.

The resources for dealing with these problems are infinitely greater than before. As of 2005 there were twenty-two health center organizations in the state.[24] One of them developed from Robert Smith's burgeoning private practice in Jackson and boasts an additional clinic on the campus of Tougaloo College.

There is the Jackson Medical Mall with all its services, and there are private programs that didn't exist thirty years ago. One of these is an interfaith church-based project called Stewpot Community Services, after the group's tradition of providing a daily meal. Located in a poor, run-down area of West Jackson, Stewpot serves a largely single and adult population with multiple, often severe, problems. It rehabs houses, plants community gardens, operates shelters, and provides substance abuse and mental health services. St. Dominic's Health Services sponsors an on-site free primary health care clinic directed by Sister Trinita Eddington, O.P. Sister Trinita gave up a longtime career as vice president for nursing at St. Dominic's to train as a nurse practitioner and care for patients in the community. Specialty services are provided by referral arrangement with the mall. Many of the people she sees are chronically ill, require labor-intensive care (11,000 visits annually for 2,000 patients), and have little hope of changing their lives. Others, she says proudly, have gotten jobs and returned to families they had left.[25]

The men and women responsible for a virtual health care revolution in Mississippi are hopeful. Their belief in the responsibilities of individuals and society is strong. Yet they question the next generation's will to address today's issues. For example, Helen Barnes is concerned about young people's motivation. Described by Jack Geiger as "the closest thing to Pearl Bailey," the husky-voiced jazz singer, Barnes has white hair now. In charge of primary care/women's health for the University Medical Center at the mall, her office is filled with mementos, from a photo of a sad-eyed woman with a homemade wooden leg and her toddler, to a formal, autographed picture of her Kings County Medical Center mentor, Louis Hellman, whose gynecology text is still in use.

During our conversation, Barnes pauses frequently to counsel the residents she is training. She explains that she holds them to high standards, not only medically but in terms of attitude and behavior as well. "All my residents call their patients by their surnames," she explains. "My grandmother taught me to treat and speak to people the way you want to be spoken to—and that you can do anything anyone else can do and, with a little effort, do it better." Families need to recognize that they are the best way to change society, Barnes believes. "We always talked and ate together at the dinner table. That's the beginning of teaching the value of discipline. You need it to do math, reading, homework. Young people need to see that change is necessary, but also that it's quicker and better to be part of it."

L. C. Dorsey is currently employed at Mississippi Valley State University in the Delta, where her first work assignments were to preserve black history and find opportunities for economic development. She is now a professor in the department of social work. The university, once a "separate but equal" showplace, has broad avenues named for civil rights legends. The campus is lined with deep pink crape myrtle, oak, and magnolia trees. Dorsey says they remind her of the trees she planted when she was director of the Delta Health Center. Slender and pretty, she's as feisty as ever. She, too, would like to see people take more responsibility for each other, in ways that range from a more generous and humane welfare program to one of her current crusades— opposition to the marketing of fast food as the only way to be healthy.

If you visit Aaron and Ollye Shirley on the right night you might get a seminar in grassroots action. They have a few friends over to their comfortable home in Jackson, and the friends just happen to be the movers and shakers who tell you how it is in Mississippi, and what they are doing to make it better. Stylish and decisive, Ollye Shirley is in charge of services to youth for a national group of mostly black women known as The Links, where she reviews the reports of some 200 local groups and helps distribute funds to them. She's also the education chair for the Mississippi NAACP. The Shirley children are all dedicated civil rights workers, she says, but too few others are involved. "We have to figure out how to mobilize people today. They're out there making money and they don't give a damn. Even if you take a higher job, you are your brother's keeper. You didn't get here by yourself."

Aaron Shirley went on to become a member of the prestigious Institute of Medicine and to serve as a health policy adviser to Bill Clinton. In 2004 he was appointed as one of fourteen members of the Citizens' Health Care Working Group, established by Congress to create a "national dialogue" on health services. There's something of the statesman about him, yet he's happy cooking catfish at home for friends and family and discussing the state of the world. "The whole universe has moved, but the gaps are still as great," he says. "We're starving social programs while we pour money into private prison systems with all the wrong incentives. Black professional women have a hard time finding men of like mind and passing on their hard-won gains to their children."

Aaron Shirley describes a recent trip through the neighborhood he grew up in. "It reminded me of a banana left out in the sun. The kids were running around half naked, barefoot. A bunch of adults were ignoring them, smoking and drinking. It's no place for people to live. We saw similar stuff in the sixties when we were documenting hunger and poverty," he recalls. "Then it was enforced by law, politics, and economics. But if anyone offered a glimmer of hope, people responded. Now it's enforced from within." The family support, the community structures, the little stores are all gone, Shirley says. "No one's raising the kids, much less reading to them and teaching them how to behave when they get to school." It's got his attention, though, and he wants to contact area parents and start a truancy prevention program.

Still making lemonade from lemons, he's working with the state to involve health centers in reducing Medicaid costs and improving services. Mississippi has come some distance since it was one of the least generous states in the country. In 2004, 19.9 percent of its nonelderly people were uninsured—more than the national average of 17.8 percent but a lower rate than in eight other states. And 38.2 percent of its nonelderly poor and near poor were uninsured, compared with a national average of 40.6 percent.[26] But Medicaid services are in danger of being cut in a way that would adversely affect beneficiaries. Instead, Shirley would like to promote better management of maternity care and conditions like hypertension and diabetes. He's also interested in better ways of dealing with patients who show up at hospital emergency rooms for nonurgent purposes. On one particular day, Shirley is hopping mad about a computer printout that reveals a pattern of inappropriate (and expensive) emergency room use by the patients of one health center he won't name. The problem, he says, is that the doctors go home at 5 P.M. and aren't available until the next day.

Almost wistfully, he harkens back to the early days when he and his partner had day and evening office hours, drove to Mound Bayou and back, and still took emergency calls every other night. "Andy wouldn't think of not being available," Shirley says. "He had more patients, and more hospital visits, than any doctor I've known since. If a patient showed up at either of our homes, our wives wouldn't dream of not inviting them in."

So now it's really about lasting ties between old friends and partners, forged in the fire of a cause far stronger than any recent rift. Despite their disagreement over the mall, Shirley visits Anderson every week, solicitous about his health problems. And Anderson, a commanding presence as befits an ex-football player, is quick on the draw when he speaks of the good times—and quick to praise Shirley for all he has accomplished. "Aaron was the main person," he says. "A heck of a guy for developing things." Anderson remembers when the two of them would debate the merits of a new scheme, with the center's social worker as a referee. "Then we'd go to the Kitty Kat and get us a drink of whisky. By the time we finished the problems were solved."

Chapter 3

Boston:

The Way Democracy Ought to Work

It's early morning in East Boston, a polyglot peninsula surrounded by water and cut off from the rest of the city by Logan Airport and its feeder roads. Jack Cradock is standing at the entrance to the health center he runs, along with medical director Jim Taylor. Since 9/11 they've made a practice of starting the day this way. It seems to remind them of why they are there and to remind the people of the neighborhood—including a sizable Arabic population—that the center is there for them.

Boston, after all, is a city of neighborhoods—a tradition that runs from the villages of colonial days to Brahmin enclaves and then to the densely populated gateway communities of the last 150 years. Points of view differ, and so does the way they are expressed, through town meetings, discussions of lofty democratic ideals, or the give and take of ward patronage. House of Representatives Speaker Tip O'Neill once famously said all politics is local, and that includes the politics of health care. Which helps explain why Boston is home not only to the first health center in the U.S. but also to more centers than any other city.

Death Zones and Vanishing Doctors

This book describes several places where poverty exists cheek-by-jowl with great affluence. In Boston, before there were health centers, there was also a crying need for care in the shadow of three great medical schools. Low-income neighborhoods had desperate health problems. One of the worst was the South End. One health center leader remembers that the *Boston Globe* described it as a "death zone."[1] Tris Blake, director of the center that serves the area today, points to an old graveyard with only a few stones. "You'd be surprised to know that 40,000 people are buried there," he says. "This was the mass grave for victims of cholera and typhoid epidemics. It's solid ground, not landfill like much of downtown. Wagons would come here and unload the bodies. Then it became an entry point for new arrivals, which meant crowded tenements and brownstones converted to rooming houses with twenty to thirty people in each." As recently as the sixties, Blake reports, "there were rats, lead poisoning, infectious disease and the highest mortality rate in Boston—all within a few miles of every major teaching hospital."[2] In 1965 the infant mortality rate in the South End was 42 deaths per 1,000 live births, compared with 24 for the city of Boston and 24.7 for the U.S. The death rate from tuberculosis was more than six times that of the city as a whole.[3]

Working-class areas were affected, too. Despite one of the nation's highest physician-to-population ratios, Boston's private practitioners had retired or had abandoned the neighborhoods. In 1940, 65 percent of the city's doctors had their offices in the community; in 1961 a phenomenal 60 percent practiced in hospitals.[4] In the blue-collar North End, nearly 70 percent of births were to women who lacked timely prenatal care, compared with a national figure of 32 percent.[5] In another neighborhood, 40 percent of people with chronic conditions like diabetes, hypertension, or heart or kidney disease went untreated.[6]

Despite racial strife, blacks, whites, and Hispanics shared a dependence on outmoded, hard-to-reach, fragmented, and disrespectful charity care, most often at Boston City Hospital (BCH). Jean Hunt, a nurse who helped organize several early health centers, recalls: "There were no doctors in my neighborhood. Stuck without a car, young mothers had to take three different trains and buses to the only source of care, wrestling the baby carriage on and off each one. When you finally reached BCH you had to wait hours in a big cold hall on hard benches. You rarely saw the same doctor twice, but then you didn't want to because they were so rude."[7]

Others shared her view: "I trained at BCH, spent 1963–1965 and 1968–1970 there. I saw the fifteen rows of wooden benches, residents seeing patients without charts. It was a pretty awful health care system," says one physician.[8] And a member of the hospital board observes: "You never saw such miserable people. It was like something out of Dickens."[9]

Marsha Barros, a health center patient and early board member, remembers: "There was this one nurse at BCH who was mean and hateful to black people. One time a moped had hit me, cracked my pelvis. The ambulance took me to BCH. I said I wanted to go to another hospital. That nurse pushed me so hard I nearly fell out of the wheelchair."[10]

Inpatient care was notoriously disorganized, according to Herbert Gleason, who later helped the city reform its health services. "BCH wards were private fiefdoms of the three medical schools—Harvard, Tufts, and Boston University, or BU. Each had its own staff. Patients were 'teaching material' assigned to a particular school on a strict rotation system. So at any given time you could have patients lined up in the hall waiting to get into a full unit while others were nearly empty because you couldn't put a Harvard patient on a BU ward."

More generally, Boston faced rapidly changing demographics, deterioration of business districts, and decaying housing stock.[11] The standard remedy was urban renewal, which usually involved invoking eminent domain, razing the entire neighborhood, and erecting modern buildings without stores, meeting places, and all the other things that make a community home. The South End had lost two-thirds of its population in the previous twenty years and was about to lose many who remained. "Villages were being destroyed," according to Blake, "and nothing will get a Boston resident as angry as the thought that his neighborhood is in harm's way."

Some of the worst pathology—ultimate testimony to what was wrong with urban renewal—was found in public housing projects. One of them, Columbia Point, had 6,000 people in low-rise buildings on an isolated spit of land once used as a prisoner of war camp and then as a garbage dump. It was about to become the site of the nation's first health center.[12]

Columbia Point

Mississippi is the touchstone of the health center movement, the place that inspired civil rights activists to lay down the principles for a new way of delivering care. But Massachusetts is actually the first state to have an operating center.

Jack Geiger and Count Gibson, the physician-activists from Tufts medical school, had first gone to the federal Office of Economic Opportunity (OEO) with their plans for a center in the rural South and were starting to prepare a formal proposal. Geiger recalls how Columbia Point got into the mix: "Count and I realized that if Tufts went to Mississippi we were sure to be asked what we were doing 1,500 miles away when there were sorely neglected black neighborhoods close to home. We decided to try for a site in Boston as well." The Tufts department of preventive medicine had fourth-year medical students doing home visits in Columbia Point. They had surveyed a sample of 1,500 people in 500 numbered apartments and found many with unmet needs. Epidemiology was an important part of the health center model, and from that point of view, Geiger says, the site looked perfect. There were no practicing physicians and no direct transportation to sources of care. The project was four miles from several major hospitals, but visits to them and back took an average of six hours, including travel and waiting time.

"We didn't really look elsewhere," Geiger continues. "Tufts had existing ties to Columbia Point, the population seemed to fit the need profile, and the Boston Housing Authority promised to help us renovate two or three apartments." Once the grant from OEO was approved, in June 1965, there was nothing to stop the center from opening its doors six months later. It was overwhelmed with demand. By some accounts, as many as 200 patients per day received services. People came in for basic medical care and got more than they bargained for, including psychological intervention for young mothers and teams of doctors and other health professionals focused on problem families.

Unlike in Mississippi, where funding delays allowed for extensive organizing, in Boston there was little time to look for the right leadership, Geiger says. "That was one reason Columbia Point never had the level of community involvement that we did in Mississippi. When you have to rely on people who are already recognized as leaders to step forward, you don't necessarily get a focus on health problems and diverse backgrounds, and you may get people who are concerned with control of jobs and influence."

Another problem was that with services limited to a single housing project, there was little room to expand or attract new leaders. And community pride was in short supply. "There was so much crime and violence that people avoided Columbia Point. Residents were ashamed to admit they lived there," Geiger recalls. Meanwhile, high demand for services continued. "Sidney Kark, the originator of community-oriented primary care I had studied with in South Africa, came to visit. He pointed out that we were investing enormous time and effort with intractable families." Gradually the center moved from a theoretical model to focus more on provision of medical care.

The federal grant from OEO also included money for research and teaching, bolstering the status of Tufts medical school and the department chaired by Gibson, now expanded to Community Health and Social Medicine. Jeff Salloway, one of several Tufts faculty members hired to study health centers, describes the atmosphere as one of excitement and commitment. He recalls that the work being done, especially by sociologist Peter New, now deceased, helped establish the emerging field of applied anthropology. New insisted that the people being studied had a right to control the application of the results, Salloway says. "In this, he taught a brand of community-based participatory research that outlived him."[13] With Tom May of the University of Oklahoma, New also coauthored a series of interviews with national health center leaders that is widely cited in the literature.[14]

However, the Tufts arrangement ultimately produced tensions. "The War on Poverty went much further than the New Deal. Instead of providing largesse to have-nots under careful strictures—social workers looking into people's lives—the poor were supposed to control the resources themselves," Salloway explains. There were combative meetings with the Columbia Point board: "Geiger was a firebrand, thoroughly charismatic, pursuing his agenda. Other faculty members tried to ferret out what the community wanted." Either way, entrenched academics weren't necessarily comfortable with the constant give and take.

In 1970 Count Gibson left Tufts for Stanford. Geiger was now directing both health centers and chairing the department. In 1971, exhausted from working three jobs and commuting between Boston and Mississippi, he announced his departure for the State University of New York at Stony Brook. "Three of the senior staff were coming with me, and the Mississippi center had indicated it was going to Stony Brook as well," he explains. "Tufts was faced with rebuilding the department and operating Columbia Point, with the board clamoring for control." Some believe that reduction of attractive overhead payments also influenced what happened. The school stood to lose indirect costs attributable to the Mississippi center. In addition, as federal administration of health centers was transferred from OEO to the Department of Health, Education and Welfare (HEW), tighter funding standards were applied. Tufts turned down the $1.4 million offered by HEW to run Columbia Point, disbanded the Department of Community Health and Social Medicine, and turned its other grants back to the funders. The remaining faculty dispersed, and sponsorship of Columbia Point shifted to Boston's antipoverty agency.[15]

A Catalyst for Growth

Despite its turbulent beginnings, Columbia Point had a profound impact on federal policy. It was located in the congressional district of then House Speaker John McCormack and the state represented by Senator Ted Kennedy, youngest brother of the slain president. Elected in 1962, Kennedy sat on the Senate Labor and Public Welfare Committee, which had jurisdiction over health issues, but he hadn't yet been identified with the topic. His August 1966 visit to Columbia Point and subsequent consultations with Geiger and Gibson led to the first dedicated federal funding for health centers and a lifelong commitment to their way of delivering services.[16] Kennedy's legislation, according to Geiger, started the process by which community groups agitated for health centers and members of Congress thought it a good idea to bring one home to their districts.

Columbia Point also served as the local catalyst for an unprecedented grassroots movement that saw eighteen more centers established in the Boston area by 1971. A newly awakened consciousness on the part of major teaching hospitals played a role. Harvard began working with activists in the Bromley Heath housing project in Jamaica Plain and received OEO support for what would become the Martha May Eliot Health Center. BU helped establish the Roxbury Comprehensive Community Health Center, also funded by OEO.[17]

Proactive development and funding by the city government affected many more areas. "The city was putting $5 million on the table," says Jim Hunt, who today heads the Massachusetts League of Community Health Centers. "But the most important factor was simply mothers seeking doctors for their kids."

In 1967 Kevin White had been elected mayor, defeating Boston School Committee chair and vociferous integration opponent Louise Day Hicks. Gleason, White's corporation counsel and also member and later board chair of the city's Department of Health and Hospitals, remembers the genesis of the city's interest in health: "BCH had always been a mess, but when we took over it really blew up in our faces. The house officers staged a 'heal in' to protest conditions, refusing to discharge patients. An aggressive reporter from the *Boston Globe* was on our case about the awful health statistics. And mothers were pushing their baby carriages around City Hall to highlight the lack of services. There was a lot of spirit in the communities, and fighting urban renewal had shown many of them they could have an impact."

In 1969 Health and Hospitals commissioner Andrew Sackett announced a "districting plan" geared toward a citywide solution. Hospitals were asked to help develop community-based centers that would provide primary medical care in specific neighborhoods and offered financial aid for doing so—matching grants for the private nonprofits or support through BCH where the city institution took responsibility.[18] The approach fit with the mayor's concept of "little city halls," decentralizing access to a whole range of services at the neighborhood level.

The Department of Health and Hospitals hired Jim Hooley to organize community support for the new centers—an unusual role for local government then and probably rarer today. Tall and modest, Hooley was known as a standout basketball star at Boston College. Drafted by the pros, he chose community work instead, and enjoyed great credibility in the neighborhoods, according to other health center leaders.

"I grew up in a housing project in Roxbury; went to the settlement house myself," Hooley says. "I wanted to build on local leadership. All of the centers provided basic primary medical care. But in the North End, for example, two additional services we provided were podiatry and dentistry because that was what was needed by the elderly, the women, and the kids. Other neighborhoods had different needs." The medical school projects were larger and funded generously by the federal government, he explains, but they had a specific model in mind, and that didn't always translate into more community support or better management.[19]

People were eager to get involved in Hooley's efforts. "We were bombarded with requests from people who wanted community health centers," Gleason remembers. In some places, health committees were drawn from other areas of civic action and militancy. Church leaders, academics, and health professionals were all interested. "Neighborhood leadership was so complicated the average person can't comprehend it today," Hooley says. "We provided training for the consumers through the city antipoverty agency. I'd go to the community and do a survey; tell them they were arming themselves with information that professionals wouldn't have when they negotiated with them. It gave them confidence. In the North End we gave out 1,500 note cards with questions. In two weeks we got 1,300 back."

Hooley continues: "Then we would find an institutional setting—a settlement house or church—to establish committees and hold meetings. I remember that one guy from North End Settlement brought a bunch of health professionals to a meeting. I asked him to go back and get the mothers—they were the key. One of them, Elaine Wilson, ended up as board chair. Her son had daily asthma attacks, and one of her goals was to have an x-ray machine in her neighborhood."

In the south Dorchester neighborhood of Neponset, one leader was afraid of speaking out. "We wrote her speech out together," Hooley remembers. "It wasn't that sophisticated but it was genuine—and very successful at convincing the professionals of what was needed." Jean Hunt, one of the Neponset mothers, says, "I learned more from those community action experiences than from the two graduate degrees I've earned."

A lot went into setting up the new facilities. In some areas, there were relief stations that could be converted to use as primary care centers. Many neighborhoods had buildings originally donated to the city by the George Robert White family for education and recreation. Others rented storefronts. Community activists and their families pitched in with carpentry and paintbrushes. Retired doctors lent their office furniture. "We ended up with ten to fifteen centers in just a few years," says Hooley.

One Neighborhood at a Time

Jim Hunt is doing something he clearly relishes—mapping the explosion of health center growth on the big greaseboard in his conference room. Points grow into circles and the circles expand, amoeba-like. Eventually the whole city is covered. It's not just a single story—there's one for every neighborhood. Four of them provide a good sampling of the similarities and differences among the communities and the centers they developed.

Roxbury

Roxbury was and is Boston's largest black community, and home to the health center with the largest federal investment. The Roxbury health service commit-tee actually began working in 1964 to bring better health care to residents. One member was Marsha Barros, a ladies' garment worker who had come to Boston from Georgia twenty years earlier. "In 1967 we were having a meeting, and a doctor who had been involved in Columbia Point and Mississippi suggested that we start a community health center," she remembers. "He helped us write the proposal. BU was the umbrella. They had a bad reputation in the com-munity—fences everywhere—and they were trying to reach out. We were shocked that the feds gave us a grant as quickly as they did. There was nothing in place, and at first we had to give the money back."

The following year the program began providing prenatal care to preg-nant women and health services to children. Then, Barros says, "we got a space in one of the old White buildings, a board, some people who knew about health." In 1969 the Roxbury Comprehensive Community Health Cen-ter, Roxbury Comp for short, formally opened its doors. "Patients came right away," according to Barros. "Like me, they were just so happy to have some-place to go where you could be treated like a human being. Other centers that followed came to Roxbury to learn how we did it. The next year we got $2 million."

What about charges that the center was overfunded or mismanaged by BU? Barros responds: "When the health center movement was young they were throwing money at it. But that was good—a lot of people who didn't finish high school got degrees, and jobs." Barros herself hired on as a community health worker at the local mental health center BU had also helped to start. Then, she says, "I got a BA in psychology and social work at BU—I never would have done it if not for the movement. It was a struggle, but still fun. Roxbury Comp had a paraprofessional training program for community residents. A lot of little people got raised up by the health center movement. It goes to show you can change things."

Over time, Barros recalls, "The feds did get more stringent with health centers—a whole lot of regulations. It made us better watchdogs. Most of the time something good came of it." She served on the health center board for twenty years, including a stint as chair. The early meetings were tempestuous, she remembers. "A lot of them were held at my house, hiding from disruptive people." The board had started with advisory status, but in 1973 control shifted from BU to the community. Later in the seventies the center underwent a major expansion and built the large modern facility it occupies today.

South End

The health center that developed in Boston's South End was like Roxbury Comp in the strength of its community roots, but in most other ways it was diametrically opposed. It started on a shoestring without institutional sponsorship or federal grants. Despite serving a large proportion of uninsured, it operated more like a private group practice, billing public and private insurance long before most centers did so. The mixed-race, heavily Hispanic community vowed to do things their own way, led by three fiercely independent men who were as different from each other as they were from some in the movement. Gerald Hass, a native of England who trained at London's prestigious Great Ormand Street Hospital, was chief of ambulatory pediatrics at BCH, charged with reorganizing outpatient services and helping to start community-based health centers.[20] Mel Scovell was a successful shoe store executive who wanted to do something different with his life when a physician friend suggested working with Hass at BCH. "I knew about retail," he explains his early contribution to the joint effort. "People come right into shoe stores—they don't need appointments. I could see that the barriers in health care had been manufactured out of the arrogance of providers, insisting on compliant patients who spoke their language."[21]

Hass and Scovell began to meet with several communities that relied on BCH, but they gravitated to the South End, where a group of mostly Hispanic men and women was spearheading health center development. As plans for the center jelled, the South End group formed a board and decided to hire Hass as medical director and Scovell as provisional executive director, with the intent of training a community resident to assume the latter post. "I was delighted with the idea," Scovell says. "But I never thought it would be a white guy."

The white guy, Tris Blake, was chosen by the community board from twenty candidates. He says race was never an issue. "We had all worked together as activists." More specifically, during the campaign against urban renewal, board members had seen Blake and his wife stand up to an armed landlord and the police. They went to jail rather than give in. Blake describes himself as a young man as someone with a "shaky education and upbringing," dropping out of high school and marrying as a teen. He and his family moved to the South End in hopes of supporting an experimental school with a diverse population, and wound up involved with housing and health. Many of the same people were active in all three, Blake says, and the city wanted to placate those inflamed over urban renewal with the promise of a health center. "First they gave us a little seed grant, space in a library, a public health nurse."

The city representatives weren't happy, however, when they learned that the South End board wanted to incorporate as the grant recipient and hire their own leaders—functions assumed by hospitals in the city's grand plan. "They were providing the money, and they said you couldn't give financial responsibility to a community board. Everywhere else, the boards had only advisory powers," recalls Scovell.

Blake, Scovell, Hass, and the South End board sat in at Health and Hospitals meetings three times. Finally, there was a negotiation over independence. Hass recalls: "It was a wonderful evening. Hundreds of people attended in a dark basement on Shawmut Avenue, and out of it came support for our approach." Tipping the balance was another key actor—city attorney Herbert Gleason.

Gleason, a patrician-looking Boston Brahmin, says he had learned the importance of community ties several years earlier when he fired a popular black leader from his job at United South End Settlement. "People demonstrated at my house on Beacon Hill, calling me a racist," he says. During this period, many white liberals had withdrawn from community involvement after similar experiences. Gleason learned from his confrontation and came away more, not less, committed. He put that commitment to work when confronted with the decision about South End's independence. "I had the clout to speak for the mayor. I said, 'Let's give it to them.' We worked out a compromise, and South End got a 'no strings' grant from the city that did not require hospital sponsorship. It was the best decision I ever made," Gleason declares. "South End became the model for the health center movement in Boston. Eventually most health centers were given the same option."

The South End Community Health Center opened its doors in May 1969 with a staff of four, including a nurse from BCH and a social worker paid for by the local tuberculosis association. Outreach and social services were provided by the South End Neighborhood Action Program. At first the center focused on medical services for children. "They poured in," Hass remembers. "I knew many of them from the BU home visiting program. There were 500 kids who were supposed to go to camp and needed physicals and immunizations. We rounded up docs and medical students. Those kids and their families became the nucleus of the health center."

Another innovation was finding an independent revenue source. According to Blake, "Mel Scovell's master stroke was to seek reimbursement from Medicaid, the federal-state insurance program for low income people, on our own. He thought if private doctors could do it we could, too. We went to the welfare department to get a license, and to the state rate setting commission. The first rates were $8.75 for a pediatric visit and $12.60 for obstetrics. Mel's family did the billing around the kitchen table, with borrowed equipment from BCH." "Everything was personal," Scovell recalls. "I would take piles of claims forms to the welfare office myself. The key to getting paid was to find your way to the desk of Honora Kelly."

Building on pediatric services, South End got space for expansion in 1975 and began providing primary care to patients of all ages. In 1980 it was cited as one of three models in the country for provision of outreach and bilingual services to Hispanics.[22] In 1985, according to Blake, the center was asked to assume responsibility for outpatient mental health services, which grew to one-third of their business.

East Boston

East Boston's background as a gateway community is evident from an old mural on the building facing the center's main entrance. One panel, "The History of East Boston Immigration," depicts Irish, Italians, American Indians, English, Latin Americans, East European Jews, and Canadians. A second, "The History of Our Block: A Community of Caring," shows area churches and synagogues. Prior to 1970 the neighborhood also featured city-sponsored health services for low-income people, including a "relief station" or emergency facility staffed by nurses and residents from BCH, and some dental, well-baby, and obstetric care in one of the city's George Robert White buildings. In the late sixties, city representatives met with the antipoverty agency for East Boston and the local group opposed to airport expansion to work on consolidating the city health services and supporting full pediatric and adult care.[23]

Logan Airport loomed large as an organizing factor, helping to isolate the community and threatening to take even more land. At one point mothers marched to protest construction on the airport expressway, pushing their baby carriages in the way of trucks, according to Jack Cradock. "It was harder in East Boston than in some other places that already had health activists," Jim Hooley recalls, but a board was eventually formed.

Jim Taylor had trained at BCH and then gone off to study cholera in Bangladesh. "Based on that experience I got interested in community health, and when I returned to BCH as senior resident I started working with the East Boston group. I liked that people from the city were interested in organizing the community and holding the hospitals responsible." The East Boston Neighborhood Health Center opened its doors in March 1970. "We had pot luck funding and part-time staffing," Taylor recalls. "One pediatrician commuted from Providence, Rhode Island. We used residents from BCH and took the bloods there for testing. The administrative structure was loose; nurses helped put the pieces together."

"In 1971 I became medical director," Taylor continues. "I was still being paid on a grant from the National Institutes of Health for hypertension follow-up." There was rapid growth, fueled in part by research and outreach on hypertension and urinary tract infection. The center acquired its own administrative staff, but space was at a premium. "We burst our building within a year," Taylor recalls. While East Boston received no operational funding from OEO or HEW, they put together an application for the federal Hill-Burton health facilities construction program in 1973. The community voted to give all of its community development block grant money for the required match.

In 1975, after having incorporated as a nonprofit organization on its own, the East Boston board was looking for an executive director. They chose Cradock, another health center legend who exchanged his business career for a value-driven vocation.

Sandy haired and soft-spoken, Cradock had worked for Raytheon and Johnson and Johnson after college. He and his wife moved back to their old neighborhood in Jamaica Plain at the end of the sixties. Calling themselves the "new urban guerrillas," they reaffirmed their commitment to a racially troubled city, supporting school busing and community services. "Moving back was in keeping with our own faith and beliefs—a perfect way for us to live our values," Cradock recalls. "My wife, Susie, a nurse on the local health committee, asked me along to a meeting and pretty soon I was hired at age twenty-six to start a center in the Brookside area of Jamaica Plain, funded mostly through the federal Housing and Urban and Development Model Cities program," he explains. "We started with a bunch of trailers circled like wagons in a church parking lot, down the street from where I grew up."

In 1974 Cradock took a year off, caring for people with polio and the elderly in a small settlement house on the California-Mexico border. When he returned to Boston, he did a brief stint as temporary director of the South Cove Health Center in Chinatown and then went on to head the East Boston center. "I was impressed with this neighborhood's straight, unpretentious working-class people and the commitment of staff," Cradock remembers. "And Jim Taylor had already put in place the philosophy I shared."

The East Boston center added home care and other programs for the elderly; reorganized the relief station into a twenty-four-hour emergency room; and turned confrontation into collaboration by negotiating with the airport to provide its emergency services. It seemed as if no addition or expansion was too daunting. When the new facility finally opened in 1978, Cradock says, "It was a major turning point. We were no longer just a poverty clinic." Also serving elderly and blue-collar residents, the center collected Medicare, Medicaid, and private insurance payments through arrangements with cooperating hospitals. Later it took on some federal operating funds, although the HEW health center program never provided a significant portion of its budget.[24]

Neponset

The neighborhood of Neponset occupies one corner of South Dorchester—until recent years, a stronghold of the Irish working class. Its residents were public employees, laborers, utility workers, truck drivers, and restaurant and retail workers. In the late sixties, several groups of local residents concerned about the lack of doctors and inaccessibility of outpatient facilities formed a health committee.

Jean Hunt, a passionate health center board member even today, remembers: "We came together as a group, met in local homes. Then we presented our issues to the local hospital. They offered us a little van, which was not acceptable. Then we met with representatives of the city who were interested in starting a health center." She continues: "Those were fun days. People were able to overcome barriers, identify needs, and solve problems. It was the sixties. People in my community thought we were lefties. There was distrust early on, but that soon changed when they became active patients."

The Neponset Health Center, funded by the city through a matching grant to Carney Hospital, began operations in a small storefront in December 1970. The board incorporated and was licensed as a freestanding clinic. At first the center open just a few sessions a week. Then in 1971 it also received federal funding through HEW, enabling it to expand space and services. In 1974 it obtained a federal Hill-Burton grant for a new building, matched by community development block grant money and its own savings. And in 1977 the center moved to the new facility—the same one it occupies today. At the board's insistence, the building was designed with separate waiting rooms for each service to avoid the look of a charity clinic.

Poised for major growth, Neponset sought an executive director familiar with the health center world. "Our first director was a young hospital administrator. We said we'd supply the street smarts. The second was similar," Jean Hunt recalls. Then Dan Driscoll arrived. He was almost a native son, born in Dorchester, but early on his parents had moved to a nearby community. Interested in city planning, he enrolled for his master's degree at Cornell in 1972 and got involved with health centers to satisfy his financial aid fellowship. His thesis topic was the War on Poverty and its doctrine of maximum feasible participation of the poor. "It seemed to me that while the centers were born out of the rhetoric of community participation, they were dominated by medical schools and professionals," he notes. He visited several health centers, spoke with Jack Geiger and Count Gibson, and decided to focus on the Tufts–Columbia Point power struggle. After graduate school, Driscoll worked as a city planner in Quincy, focusing on social services and serving as president of the local OEO agency. He spent two years at the state health center association and took the political know-how he gained there to Neponset, where he developed a reputation for good management and carefully planned expansion.

Driscoll is pleasantly noncynical about his role, the wise-guy attitude in his thesis burnished off by experience. "I came to work as a missionary, but found people didn't want to be saved," he says. "Their goals for themselves and their families were much more basic—day-to-day stuff. They weren't wearing work shirts and granny glasses. They wanted the damn services." He adds: "The last of the young mothers who organized Neponset worked here until 2004, along with two more generations of her family."[25]

The Power of Joint Action

In 1971 representatives from Boston's health centers and other agencies attended a meeting at Northeastern University intended to promote collaboration in public health planning. Their discussions also focused on issues of funding and survival, resulting in formation of the Massachusetts League of Neighborhood (later Community) Health Centers the following year. As centers outside Boston were identified or established, they were added. Marsha Barros of Roxbury was one of the health center patients and board members who helped found the league. "Someone came up with the idea that we needed a trade association. Three or four of us sat in a hotel room and wrote the bylaws. We were incorporated before the national association."

Early on, the Massachusetts League had a total of three directors in six years. It focused mostly on mutual self-help for center administrators. Jim Hunt started as a volunteer in 1974, and signed on as health resources director in

1977. Mel Scovell from the South End was interim director, grooming Hunt for the leadership position. When Hunt took over in 1979, he was twenty-eight years old.

Growing up in Neponset, Hunt had knocked on doors for local candidates from the time he was fourteen and was determined to make a career in community-based politics. After high school, he went to work for the city Department of Public Works—standard practice in a neighborhood that valued job security and longevity above most other factors. Hunt's first experience with health care was helping his wife, Jean, paint exam rooms for the Neponset center. Then he helped address personnel, zoning, and licensure issues, and it was a natural step to aiding other centers. The erstwhile volunteer became the main driver of the health centers' political success. "He pulls rabbits out of the hat and keeps pulling them," says one center director. But first Hunt had to get the disparate centers together.

The city was deeply polarized. In the best of times Boston's neighborhoods collaborated only when they had to. In the mid-seventies, people were barely talking. Separated by geography and race, they had just been through the worst of the school busing wars. For years, black activists had fought for school integration, frustrated by an unresponsive elected school committee chaired by Louise Day Hicks. Finally, they filed a lawsuit, culminating in implementation of Judge Arthur Garrity's controversial plan to bus black and white students into each other's neighborhoods. Boston is small and its geographic confines very tight, so the impact of busing students was felt primarily in a few communities where the poor and the near poor were fighting each other over diminished resources. Violent confrontations followed; it wasn't the city's finest hour.

There were also historical and philosophic differences among health centers. Hunt says: "There's an irony about the growth of centers. They built on the demands of ordinary people and continued to use the neighborhood power structures that had always defined Boston politics, but that was both a strength and a weakness. The neighborhoods had spirit and independence but they were also isolated and competitive, even jealous."

It probably didn't help that, early on, OEO had targeted the poorest neighborhoods with the highest number of minorities with its generous, holistic job-creation model, and that many of the homegrown projects in white working-class areas had less, if any, grant funding and a narrower focus. While there were exceptions, it was hard for white working-class centers not to be resentful, and equally hard for poor, predominantly black centers to accept critiques of waste and inefficiency.

"It took a long time to build trust among consumers and trust of me," Hunt remembers. "People were brought to tears on a regular basis; the word 'racism' was commonly used as a proxy for frustration. It wasn't as easy as I thought it would be. There were strong personalities, and pressures not to play in the system, to be militant. We were successful when we were focused on a common opportunity—or a common enemy—and turned the energy to collective action." Barros remembers that period well. "We had good leaders," she says. "Jim was a peacemaker. There were incidents that put him on the spot, could have meant a blowup, but he was even handed."

Gradually the centers began to function as a group. There was cross-fertilization among the neighborhoods as they found they could learn from each other. Joint action paid off, first in a cooperative assistance program for the centers building on Scovell's work. "Who would better understand a center not getting their billing done in time but someone else who had been there? There was absolute confidentiality, no such thing as a dumb question, and no fear in coming for help," Hunt says. That was the forerunner of a more formal mentoring program.

In terms of external advocacy, the Massachusetts League focused on state support. "The job was easier because we had a strong case," Hunt recalls. The league assessed the need for and effectiveness of health centers and organized clinicians and consumers to present the arguments for increased resources. Its chain of successes includes state Medicaid expansions and more generous rates for centers, grants for the centers' public health functions, establishment and participation in a state uncompensated care pool, and sharing in the proceeds from tobacco taxes and lawsuits. It also developed an analysis of health centers as "economic engines," affecting their communities by direct spending on personnel and services and doubling that sum when expenditures by local businesses are considered.[26]

Hunt notes that even with more recent budget constraints, Massachusetts invested $10 million in keeping centers financially healthy and another $21.5 million in a "campaign for excellence," including quality improvement, addition of specialists, and expansion of urgent care hours to reduce emergency room use. As of 2004 only 12.7 percent of the state's nonelderly population was uninsured, compared with the national average of 17.8 percent.[27] But the next big issue was a major effort by the state's Republican governor, Mitt Romney, and the Democratic legislature to provide universal coverage. The legislation that passed in April 2006 uses a combination of individual mandates, Medicaid expansion, and subsidized private plans to insure nearly all residents. As with most new programs, the devil is in the details, with such significant questions as plan characteristics and linkages with employers and individuals left to a new state-appointed entity known as "the Connector." According to Hunt, who is upbeat about the reforms, issues for health centers and the people they serve include whether plans will be crafted without high copayments and deductibles, and whether the combination of carrots and sticks will increase individual and employer participation. Also up in the air is the fate of the state's uncompensated care fund, which currently helps support centers and safety net hospitals but is scheduled to be diverted to the new program after 2007.

Managed Care

Managed care has been one big roller coaster ride for many health centers, and Massachusetts, with one of the first center-based plans, is no exception. Here the story seems to have a happy ending, but not without a lot of twists and turns.

In 1986, some time before managed care was fully embraced by the federal Medicaid program as the answer to rising costs, it was beginning to catch on among major players on the Boston health care scene. Jim Hunt and the health center directors found that their patients with employer-based insurance were signing up with private plans at work. The centers continued to care for these patients but could not collect payments for them. Looking for ways to stem their loss of revenues to private plans, the centers determined that the answer was their own health maintenance organization (HMO). According to Jim Hooley, who was involved in the negotiations, the centers arranged to acquire a languishing plan that city officials had tried to organize around a base of BCH patients and city workers.

Herbert Gleason, who was also involved, says, "We were finally able to spin off a health center-based HMO. We called it the Neighborhood Health Plan (NHP). Deborah Jackson from Roxbury Comp was the first chair, and Jay Harrington the first director. It began to flourish because of the health center directors on the board. It was a provider-driven plan, but these providers were in close touch with their patients."

Even so, NHP wasn't immune to the siren song of a diversified caseload. It seemed to make sense to include private provider groups, market to middle-class patients, and help other states to replicate the model. It took several years before NHP's board of center directors decided that they would do best sticking with the population they knew how to serve. In 1996 they hired Hooley, who had gone from organizing centers to running one for twenty years, as the plan's CEO. They voted to refocus on the Massachusetts centers and their patients.

The turnaround took time, Hooley explains: "Two years later we were still running a sister plan in Rhode Island, where we had lost $7 million. And we were concerned about the competition at home—big networks or provider-owned plans. We needed capital." Health center–based plans have less opportunity to accumulate the reserves other HMOs use to upgrade facilities and data systems, and they lack the deep pockets to tide them over rough spots. "Hospitals were throwing a lot of money at health centers," Hooley continues. "So we affiliated with the Harvard-Pilgrim Health Plan. They invested $5 million in NHP and established a $15 million enhancement fund to be shared among forty-two centers. But they owned us, controlling seven of the twelve board seats."

Then, Hooley says, Harvard-Pilgrim got into trouble, plunging from 1.4 million to 700,000 members, just as NHP was building its assets and controlling Medicaid costs. "We disaffiliated in May of 2002, and we're selling ourselves as the safety net plan that can do more for people. It feels much clearer now, going back to our roots." Hooley takes great pride in turning NHP back into a health center–based plan. "The issue was what's the point of a health center plan if other insurers can meet our patients' needs. I interviewed all the executive directors—what's our value, and how do we market ourselves as a new way of doing business. We converted most of the existing NHP staff to being pro–health center. The others left."

At the same time, most other plans abandoned the Medicaid market. Hunt explains: "There were fourteen HMOs serving Medicaid patients in Massachusetts in the late eighties. Now there are two. We are the largest, with 112,000 Medicaid enrollees, and we've been asked by the state to expand." In 2005, 70 percent of NHP members were health center patients, who tend to do better on cost and quality measures, with an average of four primary care visits annually. Patients of the other NHP providers—group practices and some hospital-based primary care sites—average two primary care visits per year and use emergency rooms more, according to Hooley.

Interestingly, NHP is now pioneering "broader than health care" efforts that Hooley and some of the earliest health centers espoused. For example, the HMO receives an all-inclusive capitation for patients with HIV or severe disabilities, where managed care and up-front investment can make a huge difference. "We get capitation payments ranging from $1,700 to $7,000 per person per month from the state," Hooley says. "Instead of spending 75 percent on institutional care, we spend 25 percent."

The Rest of the Story

In Boston, more than just the relationship among centers has changed. Neighborhoods are less segregated, more ethnically diverse. There are huge Asian populations, many more Hispanics, scores of other languages. Nearly every center needs some interpreters. And there are new centers aimed at specific groups—the homeless and the gay and lesbian population, for example. While the basic issues are not that different, some of the neighborhood stories have come full circle. They include a precedent-breaking eldercare program, a painful bankruptcy, modern-day entrepreneurship, and the stunning irony of an unlikely alliance.

Roxbury

Since 1999 Roxbury Comp has been headed by Anita Crawford, who grew up in the same city block as the center but spent most of her career in hospital and HMO management, including a fifteen-year stint at the giant Harvard-Pilgrim Health Plan. "I was interested in health centers, but I didn't have any preconceived ideas about them," she says. "Having worked at a well-oiled machine, I found this different and challenging. The HMO patients were nearly all commercially insured, and the services were predominantly medical. Here the patients are largely Medicaid and social issues play out in medical needs."

In 2005 Rox Comp had roughly 11,000 patients, over 80 percent of whom were black. The range of services was still expansive, including homemaking and adult foster care; HIV/AIDS counseling, testing, and treatment; behavioral health care; and a large methadone maintenance program. Crawford is proud of having brought added accountability and the use of data, rather than anecdotes, for management. The language is different, she says. "Total quality management would be off-putting, so I don't use the term. The concept of customers is mind-boggling, but patients do have the ability to shop, and we have to learn that we exist because of them."

Crawford is concerned that with changing financing, it's harder to hold the bottom line, and banks are pushing health center mergers, which could be counterproductive. However, she's also optimistic enough to think about a new facility. "We've been in the same building since the 1970s," she explains. "We needed a facelift and did some renovations, but I'd like to do more."[28]

South End

The South End center took entrepreneurship a giant step further than most by redeveloping a whole city block—a $30 million undertaking including thirty-nine condos, office space, a pharmacy, cafés, green space, and, of course, a new health center facility. Tris Blake explains that they were able to expand with help from the federal Housing and Urban Development empowerment zone program as well as $3 million they raised in a capital campaign. The new housing is all "market rate," with the health center getting half the profit to subsidize its new building.

Now, he says, the yuppie revival of the South End neighborhood has brought a new set of problems. "We were a welcoming community. You could tell by the shelters and soup kitchens. I lived here for thirty years—it's a family. But the new residents claim there are too many social services. They came to a meeting with color-coded maps showing homeless programs, schools, churches. It seems like they may have defeated their own purpose, because what they showed was that we still have needs. Affordable housing is a huge issue for us now. We don't look low income any more."

Indeed, the neighborhood now has wide streets, lots of rehabbed brownstones, and community gardens. Blake reports that the bulk of South End's patients are still Hispanic, but some live elsewhere and return for care. The center is looking at more outreach, especially to the gay and lesbian population. The new building is designed around a central atrium. The first floor features optometry, audiology, and a craft co-op run by women in the community; the second has obstetrics, pediatrics, adult medicine, and records. Mental health and dental services occupy the third floor. Blake's office is open, with glass on two sides so you can look out and down. "I shared a tiny office with Dr. Hass for years, and I'm used to instant communication," he explains. "The social factor is important in design."

The three who did it their way say the health center is the most satisfying part of their work. At the end of 2005, Hass was still taking care of kids after thirty-seven years—some the grandchildren of his original patients. He's routinely written up as one of the city's best pediatricians. Mel Scovell drops in to offer advice to people who believe he provided the best training in the world. He's made a career of grooming others, without having to be in charge himself. And Blake believes that the center is able to survive primarily on insurance payments because it keeps costs below established rates. To this day it receives no direct federal operating grants for medical care. "The standard is whether you produce for the community—if you don't you're a bum in your own ballpark."

East Boston

The second half of East Boston's story is one of continuing commitment in the face of pressures that have defeated other organizations. One the one hand, the center responded to a diversifying and aging population with a pioneering program for the elderly. "We had been providing comprehensive home care for elderly families who wouldn't use nursing homes," says Jack Cradock. "Then in the early eighties Medicare drastically reduced their coverage, issuing retroactive denials for things like physical therapy visits in the home. We had an unwritten contract with the 320 people we were serving. So we went to look at On Loc, the health and social service demonstration program in California that is funded as a full risk Medicare and Medicaid HMO. Fortunately the feds wanted to expand to other demonstration sites with a program known as PACE."

Together, Medicaid and Medicare pay the East Boston center $4,000 per month for each low-income frail elderly person enrolled. That compares with an average cost of $6,000 per patient per month in a nursing home. The payment covers everything needed by the 350 enrollees—one physician per hundred patients, access to fifty building aides in four housing projects, 180 staff, day care, transportation, home repairs, and assistance with bathing, dressing, and cooking. "It's the ultimate in what we stand for," Cradock says. "There's nothing more satisfying than knowing a patient who had used the health center for thirty years is still coming to the day center, living independently. And when the time comes, 90 percent of our patients die at home." East Boston has helped to replicate five similar projects in Massachusetts.

On the other hand, there is vulnerability. Even a preeminent center like East Boston can be dragged down by financial problems because it lacks the reserves to deal with managed care reverses and Medicaid mistakes. "The late nineties were a time of competition and growth," Cradock explains. "We doubled the size of our health center; we had a $70 million budget counting all our programs, a $16 million building, electronic medical records. We were managing our patients in the hospital, and the hospital-based HMOs pushed us to assume full risk just as the reimbursement system was cutting back. By 1998 we had $5 million in debt from managed care, and we heard informally that we owed $8.2 million to the state because of an audit adjustment in the free care program."

East Boston set up an advisory committee and looked at potential budget cuts, focusing on core strengths. It closed facilities at Winthrop Hospital and Logan Airport, shut down eldercare programs in other neighborhoods, and cut 20 percent of its staff. In January 1999 the center went to bankruptcy court on borrowed funds. "People were out to get us once we looked weak," Cradock recalls. "We were the biggest single admitter in the city, and some hospitals saw an opportunity to take us over and use us as their feeder system." In particular, there was bad blood with Boston Medical Center, the system formed by the merger of BU and BCH, because East Boston had taken some of its hospital business elsewhere.

Cradock says he considered resigning, but his board gave him three unsolicited votes of confidence. The center was in and out of bankruptcy in one year. "It helped a lot that the Medicaid director said we didn't have to pay the $8.2 million audit adjustment," he says. Two years later it was doing a little better than break even.

In 2005 the neighborhood mural facing East Boston's main entrance would have to add the Arab nations and countries from Africa and Southeast Asia to reflect the area's changing population. "Our patients speak thirty-four languages," Cradock says. "We have seventeen full-time interpreters, plus volunteers and part-timers for the rest. We are the largest employer in the community, with a staff of 800." The lesson for the future? "Always do the right thing. And after what we went through in 1999, always do the right thing carefully."

Neponset and Columbia Point

After the city poverty agency took over from Tufts as sponsor, Columbia Point broke away on its own, renaming its board the Peninsula Health Committee. It fell on hard times, many of them foretold by the community's isolation, lack of an interested backup institution, and the pathology of public housing. In 1984 the flagship center went into receivership.

Dan Driscoll of the Neponset health center, several miles to the south, recalls that Columbia Point's leaders called him the last week of that year and said the feds were going to pull their grant unless the center got new management. "They asked us to take over," he says. "It was the height of irony—a black and Hispanic community asking a white Irish Catholic group to run their center." The ironies didn't stop there. Neponset had started narrow and expanded later; Columbia Point had started broad and cut back along the way. And Driscoll, who had studied Columbia Point's early history in graduate school, would now be running it.

"At that time the housing project where the center was located had become the worst in the city," Driscoll says. "There were gangs. Fire and ambulance workers wouldn't go in without a police escort. Neponset had a board that was not only Irish and Catholic but very traditional, orderly, conservative. Yet they decided to try it for three months. The ethnic difference wasn't raised. Our consultant said Columbia Point couldn't be saved, but we were intrigued. After all, it was the first health center in the country. We overruled the consultant."

Jack Geiger says he was OK with the change in leadership. "I was much less invested in Columbia Point; never thought of it as an instrument of social change—the label that had been applied to the center in Mississippi. So the most important thing was to continue health services through incorporation into larger structure." He periodically visits the site of the original center, now renamed for him and Count Gibson, and finds the facility much improved over the early apartments they started with. Geiger is also pleased with the continued employment of community residents and the number of center doctors who are seeing their third generation of patients.

Once it was decided that the arrangement between Neponset and Columbia Point would be permanent, Driscoll remembers, they also renamed the umbrella group. "We couldn't keep the name Neponset—it meant white Catholic to everyone. The sites were on the water. So we reorganized as Harbor Health Services. We also inherited Columbia Point day care, originally intended as early intervention by the health center, but by then run separately, and a satellite in a small lily-white housing project named for Speaker McCormack's mother."

A great deal of crunching was required to create one efficiently functioning organization. Columbia Point had started with a $1.4 million federal grant that paid the lion's share of its costs. Neponset's federal grant originally covered about half of its costs. In 2005 the community health center portion of Harbor Health had a total budget of $19 million and a federal operating grant of $1.6 million. And visits to the Geiger-Gibson site were twice what they were in the mid-eighties, when the center was having its worst problems.

Integration of staff has proceeded well, but Driscoll thinks the board needs to expand its reach to include more of the changing community. "There's still a big brother-little brother dynamic, and only about 25 percent of the board is minority when it ought to be 60 or 70 percent," he admits. Despite trying to relate consumer slots to the number of patients served from each neighborhood, recruiting has been difficult. People shy away from participating, in part because some original Columbia Point board members were held personally liable during the receivership. The big problem now is gentrification.

Driscoll explains that in 1990 the housing project was completely redeveloped and renamed Harbor Point. One-third of the apartments are reserved for low-income families, which translates into roughly half the residents. The other half are young professionals paying market rates for their housing. "Now the Columbia Point area has gotten 'too good' for public housing," Geiger says. "It's home to the Kennedy Library and the University of Massachusetts. It's still geographically but not socially isolated."

Neponset's neighborhood has changed as well. The stronghold of the Irish working class has finally given way to the diversity surging across the U.S. "Language is a major issue among our 22,000 users," Driscoll reports. "We need more than interpreters. It's a question of signs, and how you answer the phone. At Geiger-Gibson the second language is Spanish. In Neponset, it's Vietnamese." But the health problems are not very different.

"So much of our resources go to treating what presents—pregnancy, diabetes, hypertension, infections, asthma. I am amazed at the amount of depression. But if you're good at public health you ask what they aren't telling you about—domestic violence, substance abuse, more depression. And then you want to know who doesn't make it to the waiting room. Before the economy in Ireland improved, undocumented people flooded into the Neponset area. We knew they were here but they weren't coming in to the center. We hired a social worker from Ireland and sent her out. First the young men came in, then the young women, then the pregnant ones. Several years later, the Vietnamese moved into the neighborhood. Our Irish social worker mentored young Vietnamese women on how to reach new immigrants. Now those who came as interpreters and outreach workers are phone operators, nurses, and accountants."

The Way Democracy Ought to Work

The fierce autonomy and unquenchable spirit in Boston's neighborhoods prompted Tom Van Coverden, head of the National Association of Community Health Centers, to observe: "It's the way democracy ought to work. America works and programs work when people are actively involved."[29] Where did that spirit come from, and why did community governance—the most controversial of health center traits, and the one most often criticized as left-wing rhetoric—take such strong root in conservative, working-class Boston?

Some of the city's health center founders would call it tradition. Others claim that the idea of community control was theirs before it was ever codified by the feds. And Herbert Gleason says: "It was a genuine effervescence. Government was open to it, but it was the people who took matters into their own hands. Jefferson thought that happiness meant influence over the decisions that affect your life. What could be more important?"

Community governance matters, from one center's board members who followed their dentist around to make sure he had enough appointments to the South End's precedent-shattering demand for autonomy. "Boards seldom make a wrong decision," says Tris Blake. "But if people are going to have their lives screwed up they may as well do it themselves."

It took a little longer, but nearly all of the Boston centers have embraced another controversial characteristic—addressing multiple factors that contribute to ill health. Even as the original OEO grantees cut back on some services, other centers that began primarily with medical care moved closer to the comprehensive model. Eventually it was Boston's neighborhoods, together with a few visionary leaders, that broadened the centers' mandates and sought new funding sources to include substance abuse, mental health, comprehensive care for the elderly and people with disabilities, housing, and even environmental interventions.

The lesson, according to Dan Driscoll: "If government can help leverage the beginnings, the community will grow the program." As far as the future is concerned, Jim Hooley says, "We're still concerned about life issues for people with no reserves for medical care or who are new to this country; how to mix community with health care interventions. Conservatives may have influenced our language but not what we are doing."

In 2005 there were twenty-five health centers in Boston and fifty-three statewide—thirty-three of them federally funded. The centers serve one in every ten Massachusetts residents, and their 677,000 patients comprise 43 percent of the state's Medicaid and uninsured and underinsured people— unusually high in an era when there are multiple actors on the safety net scene. The state and especially the city of Boston are unique in the number of centers that receive no federal funds but nevertheless follow the original health center model of comprehensive services and consumer-controlled boards.[30] Reflecting on the history, Jim Hunt says: "We're living proof that if you ask the people who are most affected, they will most likely support community governance, needed services, and a broader view of health, in that order. And if you've seen one center, that's all you've seen. Like our neighborhoods, each organization will be proudest of what makes it different."

Chapter 4

The South Carolina Low Country:

A Homegrown Black Power Structure

The stretch of Atlantic coastline from Charleston, South Carolina, to Savannah, Georgia, is a favorite of artists and writers. In what is known as the Low Country, dark trees and brush contrast starkly with wheat-colored marsh grass and wide-open skies. Close up, what seemed to be a single landscape separates into hundreds of dark channels and tiny islands. Some of the hidden coves shelter million-dollar vacation retreats and billion-dollar hotels. Others are crowded with cottages of people who work for the owners.

The transformation of this area from the home of deeply impoverished former slaves to an overheated resort and retirement economy is one story. The change from a white oligarchy to a homegrown black power structure that brought decent living conditions and state-of-the-art health care is another.

A Place Bypassed by Progress

Back in colonial times, the South Carolina Low Country boasted the nation's most prosperous plantations. Rice was a particularly labor-intensive crop, allowing for owners to maximize the economics of slavery. As recently as 1860, the ratio of blacks to whites was the country's greatest, and the state, despite its small land area, was third after Georgia and Virginia in the absolute number of slaves. With the outbreak of the Civil War in 1861, South Carolina, having been first to secede, was occupied almost immediately by Union forces. The owners deserted, leaving huge numbers of slaves to survive on their own. The Union army freed the Low Country slaves prior to Lincoln's Emancipation Proclamation, and, working with missionaries, helped provide housing, education, and employment on and near Hilton Head Island. Their efforts were called the Port

Royal Experiment, considered by some as a model for postwar Reconstruction efforts. When the soldiers decamped in 1868, three years after the war's end, the former slaves were once again left without much in the way of resources.[1]

Many survived by subsistence farming or fished from rudimentary boats. Those in the isolated outermost communities continued to speak a slave-trade dialect known as Gullah—part African and part English—and to practice traditional crafts such as basket weaving.[2]

For nearly 100 years the rural areas of the Low Country were synonymous with abject poverty, bypassed by later industrial development of the Piedmont Plateau in the western part of the state. For example, in 1960 more than 60 percent of the families in Jasper County had incomes under $3,000, rivaling places in the Mississippi Delta. This compared with 23 percent of families nationally.[3] Even as tourism came to a few of the barrier islands, others continued to lack transportation, potable water, and sewage systems. Hunger and malnutrition were commonplace, as were Third World conditions and water-borne diseases.[4]

But there were positive aspects as well. Despite prejudice and deprivation, the racial situation was not quite as bitter as it was elsewhere in the South. When the time came for change, the process was smoother. Roland Gardner, a lifelong resident of the area who today runs the health center serving the state's southeastern counties, puts it this way: "Conditions were awful and there was a lot of denial, but we didn't have the violent resistance here that they had in Mississippi and Alabama."[5]

Black land ownership was an important influence. The white plantation owners never returned in force, and former slaves were able to acquire land and make a beginning on an agrarian existence. Impoverished themselves, some of the white planters failed to pay their taxes, and their land was given to the freed slaves in ten-acre tracts. The deeds were known as "Head of Family Land Certificates," and some are still extant, signed by General William T. Sherman himself.[6] The legacy of the rice plantations was, paradoxically, a plus in its own right. There were few overseers, and slaves were left largely on their own, using cultivation methods they brought originally from Africa. Black supervisors and accountants were not uncommon; some slaves gained experience in business management and passed their knowledge on to family and friends.[7]

The isolation of the barrier islands and the sheer numbers of blacks also affected the racial climate. "Before the bridge was built there were nine white families on Hilton Head, and elsewhere you could count the number of whites on one hand," says longtime resident Tom Barnwell. "There was economic interdependence between blacks and those whites that did live here. My mother was a nurse midwife who delivered many of the white babies. And when it came to transportation, whoever had their bateaux in the channel leading out to the river would go first."

Historically, the military was a major presence in the Low Country, from the giant navy base in Charleston, now closed, to the infamous marine training center on Parris Island, near Beaufort. When the armed services were integrated, it was an example that didn't go unnoticed by local blacks as well as whites.

Another important factor was the ongoing presence of institutions dating back to the Port Royal Experiment. Chief among them was the Penn School, named for William Penn by the Quakers who came in 1862 to help educate former slaves. Located on St. Helena Island, it became the Penn Center in 1948, continuing its involvement in education and training, preserving Gullah culture and traditions, and fostering economic self-sufficiency. During the 1960s, it turned to civil rights, hosting conferences led by Martin Luther King Jr. The meetings were secretive because of criticism of King's politics and threats on his life. A Charleston television station spent a week interviewing staff and then surprised them with an "exposé" of Penn Center as a hotbed of left-wing activity. After King's assassination in 1968 there was less focus on national civil rights campaigns, and the Penn Center turned to local activism to address conditions faced by Low Country blacks.[8]

It Started with Hunger

The area's advocates rode a wave of national interest in hunger and an unprecedented series of hearings and reports. Early in 1967 Senator Robert Kennedy spearheaded hunger hearings in Mississippi, and a foundation endowed by the late department store magnate Marshall Field sent a group of physicians to report further. That led to more hearings across the country by a group known as the Citizens' Board of Inquiry into Hunger and Malnutrition, established by union leader Walter Reuther's Citizens' Crusade Against Poverty.[9]

Two figures dominate Low Country participation in these events. One, a white physician named Donald Gatch, had come from Nebraska but trained in Savannah, Georgia. After seeing the segregated waiting rooms and poor access for blacks in nearby Beaufort County, Gatch set up his private practice there. When the Citizens' Board of Inquiry came to South Carolina, he used his own experience to describe the links between malnutrition and environmental problems. Among the preschool children Gatch treated, severe anemia was widespread. Testing revealed that at least 50 percent were suffering from worm infestation, in some cases so pervasive that they were literally starving to death.[10] He also criticized the lack of care available to these children, as well as his colleagues' knowledge and complicity in allowing the situation to continue. Gatch said he tried to get help from the county health department, but it brushed his inquiries aside, telling him, "until the colored people got educated enough to wash their hands . . . there wasn't any point in treating them."[11]

While he attracted national attention from the likes of southern columnist Harry Golden writing in the *Nation*, photographer Diane Arbus, *Esquire*, and the *New York Review of Books*, Gatch was also vilified as a traitor to his own race and professional calling. His white patients left him, and his rent was doubled, so he was forced to close his office in Beaufort, losing with it his staff privileges at the local hospital.[12] State officials resented Gatch's accusations and charged him with drug violations and addiction. The situation grew heated and hostile, and, according to Barnwell, violence was threatened against the crusading doctor. Eventually the state Board of Medical Examiners dropped its charges in exchange for a plea of inadequate record keeping; Gatch lost his license, and he left the state. A courageous yet tragic figure, he was later killed somewhere in Cambodia, where he had gone to help provide medical services for refugees of the Vietnam War.[13]

The next Low Country champion had more staying power. Tom Barnwell, a fifth-generation black native of Hilton Head, had been hired by the Penn Center as director of community development. He didn't mind taking risks, and he approached his task with a kind of entrepreneurial zeal, aided by the fact that, once kindled, the spotlight on hunger continued. In 1968 South Carolina's junior senator, Fritz Hollings, held his own "hunger tours" across the state, not to be bested by outsiders. As governor, Hollings had made his mark as a moderate when he supported the integration of Clemson University, but later admitted that he downplayed poverty and hunger to attract business. "You don't catch industry with worms," he said. "Maybe fish, but not industry."[14]

That same year saw the establishment of the Senate Select Committee on Nutrition and Human Needs and the announcement of formal hearings to be held early in 1969. Barnwell was ready to go to Washington. Driving home the relationship between hunger, disease, and the environment that Gatch had established, he told the committee of his community's need for jobs, day care, housing, health care, and water and sewage treatment facilities, and of their difficulty in getting government support for these services. People on one small island, he said, routinely hauled their drinking water from a source over three miles away.[15]

Barnwell returned home to identify and organize nineteen target areas among the barrier islands of Beaufort County and the timberlands of neighboring Jasper County. Each community sent two representatives to an advisory board. One of their first acts was to change the name of the group. " 'Organiza-tion to Prevent Hunger and Malnutrition' didn't cover it," he remembers. "The issue was always broader than hunger. We became Beaufort-Jasper Comprehen-sive Health Services."

Environment and Health

However, the evolution from hunger advocacy to health care still wasn't com-plete. The organization focused first on what people saw as the most pressing needs in their communities—environmental action and home health services. It applied to the Office of Economic Opportunity (OEO) for support of a series of health-related activities and received its first grant, for $342,000, toward the end of 1969.

Barnwell was aided in his efforts by Emory Campbell, another black Hilton Head native. "I was a guinea pig, getting a masters' degree in environmental health at Tufts University in Massachusetts," Campbell recalls. "In 1970 I got the call to come back home." The first environmental services engineer in South Carolina, he headed up health education at Comp Health, as the new or-ganization was known in the community. "We mapped every house in the nine-teen target communities to figure out what was going on," Campbell continues. In addition to house-to-house surveys, local churches were a major source of information. "I never attended church as much as I did then," he says. "That's where everybody gathered."

One of Campbell's findings was widespread use of home remedies by "root doctors," including the use of herbs and drawing tea and applying sweet gum ashes to heal sores. "But," he says, "to get to the real 'root' of our problems we had to change economic and cultural habits. People had to understand the im-portance of deep wells, pumps and sanitary privies, and organize themselves to help pay for them."[16]

Barnwell established two programs to train and employ people from the area, enhancing self-sufficiency as well as health outcomes. "One group that we called community health education and action workers involved people in en-vironmental needs—proper drainage, septic tanks, shared wells," he explains. The second group, family health workers, went into people's homes to provide basic hands-on services, like caring for stroke victims. These workers received six months of intensive training, supervision by registered nurses, and in-service sessions twice a month with physicians. Eventually Comp Health became the first private home health agency certified in the state.

In 1970, four months after the first OEO grant, the organization began offering ongoing health care at a facility in Hardeeville, Jasper County, leased from the health department. Donald Gatch worked there part-time until he left the state. Today the Hardeeville site is named for him. Comp Health estimated that there were 25,000 people in the two-county area who could benefit from the physician, hospital, educational, transportation, and environmental services offered. Growth was driven not so much by health differences among the communities to be served but by the need for multiple outlying sites to accommodate the area's sixty-seven islands and roundabout roads. "Transportation was the 'Achilles' heel' of our rural preventive health care program," according to a history Roland Gardner later prepared.

The next site to open, in the Beaufort County community of Sheldon, was named for the organization's first full-time South Carolina–born physician, Elijah Washington. Washington had been released early from his obligation to the navy through the intervention of Strom Thurmond, South Carolina's other senator. A second Jasper County site was established in the community of Grays, and another Beaufort County facility, named for Leroy Browne, opened on St. Helena Island. Browne had been elected to the Beaufort County council in 1960—the first black elected to any public office in South Carolina since the turn of the century. Within two years, there were five sites and eight doctors. Although that level of growth would challenge most health care organizations, the new facilities were busy right away. "A lot of folk had never seen a doctor, and they were lined up to get in for care," Gardner recalls.[17]

Comp Health was also drawing on support from Ruth Field, Marshall Field's widow, who had provided funding for the early hunger hearings in Mississippi and elsewhere and had a special interest in Beaufort County, where she kept a vacation home and helped fund the Penn Center. She donated money to train the family health workers and five acres for the center's first permanent building in the community of Chelsea. With an additional $400,000 from OEO, construction began, and the organization's service area expanded from nineteen to thirty-two communities.

Overcoming Resistance

When it began functioning as a full-fledged health center, Comp Health faced resistance from the medical profession and Beaufort Memorial, the local hospital. The hospital had only six physicians to the center's eight. "The pervasive position among local doctors was that we represented 'socialized medicine,'" Barnwell recalls. "They were also suspicious of the physicians we had brought in. We had to challenge the hospital to get admitting privileges, and we had to reimburse them when they admitted our uninsured patients." Uninsured patients of the private physicians were admitted without such payment, but they were frequently referred back to Comp Health, whereas paying patients referred by the center were subsequently directed to the private doctors. However, things worked out in the center's favor. The hospital always seemed to need money, and the reimbursement from Comp Health helped keep it afloat during some lean years. Eventually Elijah Washington became the first black physician on Beaufort Memorial's staff.

While health services were one centerpiece, Comp Health continued to operate very much in the mode of the original, wide-ranging OEO programs. Barnwell had consulted with the early health centers in Mound Bayou and Jackson, Mississippi, and found his own creative ways to attack the environmental causes of ill health and capitalize on the potential for economic development. According to Gardner, construction of the new facility led to businesses in the community—sewage, welding, even day care and housing.

Transportation was first provided so that patients could get to the center for health care. That became the precedent for two major spin-offs. The first was a bus service to take local residents to work on Hilton Head, where there were landscaping, wait staff, and housekeeping positions in the growing tourist industry. The jobs rarely provided health insurance, but salaries were high enough to pay living expenses and even something toward medical care. The second was an emergency medical system, bringing ambulance service to the barrier islands for the first time.

"We were into economic development more than many centers," Barnwell says. Comp Health organized a food cooperative on Daufuskie Island, the least developed of the barrier islands whose name is Gullah for "the first key" in a long archipelago. "Without the co-op, residents of Daufuskie had to travel by boat to Savannah monthly for food and provisions," he recalls. Emory Campbell remembers that "some entrepreneurial efforts worked and some didn't, but we learned from all of them. A shrimp co-op failed because the participants were not schooled well enough to run it themselves. They didn't understand why selling together was a benefit."

Thaddeous Coleman's story is one of personal as well as professional success. He had been a high school teacher and assistant principal in the area for seventeen years until he lost his job to alcoholism. He got sober, joined the center's staff as special assistant for water projects, later became director of community services, and has been associated in one way or another with Comp Health ever since. "If a patient came in and the doctor determined that his illness was related to poor living conditions, there would be a referral to my department for sanitary or home repairs," Coleman recalls. The "prescription" might include installation of a septic tank or construction of a deep well to be shared by several neighbors. Families contributed on a sliding fee scale, and the remainder was subsidized. "Some years we'd put in up to seventy septic tanks," he explains. "Without this service we would have continued to have problems with worms, parasites and stomach conditions. A lot of people had shallow wells. They may have had a hog pen to one side and an outdoor privy or waste disposal to the other. You'd be drinking your own waste." The wells and septic tanks typically eliminated worms and parasites within one or two years.[18]

The next area to tackle was mental health. "The state institutions were releasing patients on meds into the community with no follow up," Barnwell says. Christmas, 1971, Roland Gardner was home on St. Helena Island writing his thesis for a master's degree in psychology from Howard University. He was not new to activism. As a high school senior, he had helped lead a boycott of the stores in Beaufort, most of which had no black salespeople. The result: the stores asked the local National Association for the Advancement of Colored People to pick black students for holiday jobs. And Gardner knew Barnwell, who had attended the Penn School and boarded nearby on St. Helena because Hilton Head had no high school.

"Tom came by my house and asked me to prepare a grant proposal for a mental health program at Comp Health," Gardner remembers. "At first I wasn't interested—I just wanted to finish school. But my mother reminded me that he had come out of his way to see me. When I got back to Washington I went over to D.C. General Hospital and worked up a proposal based on the neighborhood mental health program operating there. Several months later I was on my way to class when Tom called me from National Airport and asked me to help defend the grant at OEO. Then it was funded, and Tom wanted me to come help run it. I was still writing my thesis when I started work at the center."

Gardner came aboard as director of mental health and social services, counseling many of the patients himself. "The situation was worse than we thought," he says. In addition to schizophrenic patients discharged from state hospitals, there was a great deal of alcoholism and depression, much of it related to high unemployment and difficulties in eking out a living from fishing or truck farming. "State and county programs were not community oriented, so we got them to contract with us provide mental health, alcoholism, and drug abuse services."

In 1976 the center added another site in Ridgeland, the Jasper County seat, and a program to serve migrant and seasonal farmworkers, providing special night clinics in the summer to accommodate long work days, and transportation to and from the workers' living quarters.

A Homegrown Black Power Structure

One of Barnwell's masterstrokes was to insist that all of the health center's senior staff attend meetings of county councils; departments of health, environment, and transportation; boards of education; and other organizations that affected Low Country life. "If the meeting was held during work hours we got release time to attend," Gardner recalls. "Everyone would report back and we'd discuss how we were going to advance our agenda."

Eventually some Comp Health staffers ran for office, and others took leadership jobs in the same agencies they had been trying to infiltrate. "We developed a homegrown black power structure," according to Gardner. He notes that Louis Dore, the center's human resources director, was the first black in South Carolina to make senior partner in a major white law firm. Dore's two sons and a cousin now work at the same firm, and Dore went on to serve as chair of the state board of education. Edward Allen, director of transportation at Comp Health, became director of emergency medical services for Beaufort County and later for the state. Agnes Garvin, the center's chief accountant, became director of the county elections office. Fred Washington, the manpower director, started working at the county social services agency, eventually became its director, then served as a city councilman and mayor pro tem. And two female staffers, also center patients, became detectives in the sheriff's department.

The health care scene began to change gradually as well. Several of the physicians assigned to Comp Health by the National Health Service Corps stayed on in private practice when their terms were up, becoming part of the community. Gardner and Dore were elected to the hospital's board of trustees, where they served as active advocates for the poor—but not without initial resistance. "When we first showed up they adjourned the meeting and didn't meet again for six weeks," Gardner recalls. "Then they adopted what we called the 'Gardner rule.' Members could serve only two consecutive terms."

Gardner himself left Comp Health in 1978 to become Beaufort County's first black director of social services. "The health center gave minority individuals opportunities and helped us grow," he observes. "It strengthened the community as a whole and provided role models for young people when there wasn't much else to offer." Campbell adds: "We changed the color of government." The results included more sympathetic social services, more people enrolled in Medicaid, and better schools.

But there were some issues beyond the reach of even an enlightened and integrated local power structure. When the national management of the health center program switched from OEO to the Department of Health, Education and

Welfare, later known as Health and Human Services (HHS), many of the center's "nonhealth" activities were called into question. Barnwell made trip after trip to Washington to try to explain why he needed a backhoe to help farmers still using a horse and plow, or a barge to deliver supplies to the Daufuskie Island co-op. He failed largely because federal program officials were in the midst of a major expansion in the number of centers that required sacrifices in the scope of services.

Barnwell, ever the entrepreneur, started looking for ways to reach more people with less money and to address water and sewer problems more comprehensively. The U.S. Department of Agriculture's Farmers Home Administration (FmHA) had money to finance municipal water systems in rural areas, but it didn't want to support the smaller, community-based systems that Barnwell and Thaddeous Coleman proposed. "They thought that little communities wouldn't pay back the loans," Barnwell explains. So he and Coleman hooked up with a group called the National Demonstration Water Project (NDWP) that sued FmHA and eventually got special grant funding targeted to areas in several states. Beaufort and Jasper counties, known nationally because of the hunger hearings, were selected to receive water systems and fire protection for a number of communities, lowering insurance rates and removing a significant health threat at the same time. Eventually the NDWP expanded to other South Carolina counties, with Coleman working there full time. Barnwell continued his efforts as well, and in 1980 he took a position as regional director of the National Consumer Cooperative Bank. Roland Gardner returned to Comp Health, this time to serve as executive director. "Tom had given my name to the HHS regional office," Gardner says. "I was surprised, but he put the full court press on to convince me to come back."

Growth and Change

Early on, Gardner was faced with what he calls his greatest management challenge as director of the center: not getting fired. "The Reagan tide hit, with its funding reductions and block grant proposals," he remembers. "We took a huge cut—the staff of 200 had to be cut by more than one half, and doctors from fourteen to seven." As was often the case, some of the most innovative nonmedical services were the first to go. "We went from twelve buses to five and we could only make one trip a day. That meant that some patients had to sit in the waiting room for hours. Home health was also reduced, but luckily Tom had chartered it as a separate agency that collected Medicaid and Medicare, so many of the services were maintained." Gardner continues: "We consolidated some sites in Jasper County. I insisted on closing the facilities we didn't own and keeping the ones where we had mortgage money pending. That caused a rebellion from the communities affected—150 people came to the board meeting to protest, and I was hung in effigy. Bob Jackson from the regional office supported me. Somehow we weathered the storm and started growing back."

Comp Health rebuilt its main site in Chelsea, adding quarters for central administration and a community conference room. The health facility is named for Ruth Field, with a plaque and garden dedicated to her as the center's original benefactor. The administration building is named for Tom Barnwell, its prime mover. In 1996 the center built another large facility in Port Royal, thanks to a combination of federal and state resources, plus a bond referendum floated by the town. The $2.3 million, 22,000-square-foot elegant Spanish colonial structure is wired for electronic medical records and telecommunications, allowing for state-of-the-art research and quality improvement efforts and consultations for patients in far-flung rural communities. It's hard to distinguish from the private multispecialty group practices that line the town's main drag, known as the Medical Mile, unless you know that along with doctors' care it includes an HIV/AIDS clinic and a Women, Infants and Children feeding program.

In 2000 the center expanded inland, adding Hampton County to its name and two more sites to its growing roster. "First the health department asked us to assist with obstetric services, resulting in the Hampton site," Gardner explains. "The following year we got some of the new federal health center expansion money and purchased a private practice in Estill."

In 2005 Comp Health, now comprising eight sites and eight more school health clinics, served 19,000 patients with a staff of 178, including fourteen physicians, four nurse practitioners, and three dentists. Patients can receive medical, dental, and pharmacy services as well as home health care, and the center is now well integrated with Beaufort Memorial Hospital. It has been selected as one of ten organizations to help develop a prenatal care collaborative, similar to the diabetes effort aimed at organizing health center providers to improve services and outcomes throughout the country. The center is working with hospital staff to create cards with easily transferable information for mothers to carry when they are about to deliver, and to improve psychosocial risk assessment.[19]

Comp Health's annual budget totaled $13 million, with roughly half of that coming from public and private insurance and other patient fees—a far cry from the early days when the federal grant was the only source of revenue. Perhaps the greatest change has been in demographics. According to Gardner, a caseload that was 90 percent black, 2 percent Hispanic, and 8 percent white in 1980 has shifted to 60 percent black, 28 percent Hispanic, and 10 percent white. The center now has eleven bilingual staff members to serve the increasing number of Hispanics, drawn primarily by jobs in the burgeoning tourism industry.

In some more isolated communities, Comp Health is still providing potable water and septic tanks, but health problems have changed. In addition to HIV/AIDS, there's the "new malnutrition," something the Low Country shares with many other areas. Staff are finding obesity, diabetes, and hypertension not only among adults but also children in the center's eight school-based clinics. That could mean a new role for the center's original broader-than-health-care approach. "People have become more conscious about their health, but not about diet and exercise," explains Emory Campbell. "This was an agrarian society. People had to work to raise food. Now they're working two jobs and haven't got the time to exercise or shop and eat well. But they do have supermarkets, fast foods, microwaves and TV. They've bought into entertainment by watching, not doing."

The Larger Picture

In 2005 coastal Beaufort County, with 140,000 people, was the state's fastest-growing area, fed by tourism, agriculture, the seafood industry, and the military.[20] Hilton Head, continuing to expand, is the site of hour-long traffic backups as residents and visitors cross the single bridge from the mainland.[21] And Gardner reports that Del Webb, the Arizona developer of "Sun City" retirement communities, is building homes for 15,000 people near Bluffton, one of the last of the Low Country's pristine coastlines.

Conversely, the inland counties of Jasper and Hampton have more land but fewer people (roughly 21,000 people each) and far fewer jobs. There are major economic differences as well: the cost of a small house in Beaufort County is $140,000, compared with $80,000 for a similar property in Jasper County; the poverty rate in both inland counties exceeds 20 percent, compared with 10 percent in Beaufort County.[22] But the whole area needs better jobs, according to Gardner. "Employment on Hilton Head is mostly seasonal, still without benefits." The good news, he says, is that local residents are beginning to start businesses, and there is a possibility that the Port of Savannah, just to the south, will be dredged to allow for container shipping, with the potential for becoming the second busiest container port on the East Coast.

Health care in the area has grown, too. Beaufort Memorial Hospital had 110 physicians on staff in 2005, including all of the Comp Health doctors. There are community mental health centers serving the area, with close referral and consulting relationships to the center. And there are some additional safety net providers. Notably, a program on Hilton Head known as Volunteers in Medicine uses retired physicians under special license from the state to provide basic ambulatory care to uninsured and indigent patients. "They came to us when they were getting started and used our structure as a framework," Barnwell says. "They refer obstetrics and hospital admissions to Comp Health." The volunteer model has grown from a single clinic on Hilton Head to forty-four across the U.S.[23]

The state of South Carolina has always had some leaders like Fritz Hollings who are proud of their role in fostering the progress of Low Country blacks. On his retirement from the Senate in 2004, Hollings listed support for Comp Health and other health centers among his most important contributions. The difference is that now he's not alone. Most politicians, at a minimum, respect black voting strength. Things have improved since the years the state continually registered one of the nation's highest infant mortality rates. As late as 1986, 14 of every 1,000 babies died before their first birthday, the highest rate in the country, compared with a national average of 10.6. By 2002, 9 of every 1,000 South Carolina babies died before their first birthday compared with 6.9 for the U.S.— still high but better than several other states.[24]

Economic progress and decent sanitary conditions have helped, as has improved access to health care. In 2004, 16.8 percent of the state's nonelderly population lacked health insurance, lower than the national average of 17.8 percent.[25] Some of these gains were achieved by vigorous implementation of the State Child Health Insurance Program (SCHIP), which allows states to go beyond Medicaid restrictions to cover near-poor children.

But the huge influx of Hispanic workers, many of them not yet eligible for public insurance and some undocumented, has eaten up the gains in coverage for Comp Health. Like the state's eighteen other health centers, it is a provider of last resort for people who lack either insurance or the means to pay more than a pittance for their care. In 2000, 50 percent of Comp Health's patients were uninsured; in 2005 the figure was up to 54 percent. The federal grant continues to subsidize roughly half of the center's budget, but with the number of uninsured increasing, Gardner warns that additional dollars will be needed.

Comp Health is one of the major leaders in the South Carolina Primary Health Care Association, which provides planning and technical assistance for the centers, educates policy makers, and advocates for increased funding, improved Medicaid and SCHIP coverage, and full partnership in the state's health care decisions. Lathran Woodard, who has headed the association since 1989, knows the state scene as well as anyone. Before her current job, she worked her way up from secretary to maternal health director and then to director of administration at the South Carolina health department. A petite woman with fashion-plate looks, she loves fleshing out new policies, like special care for high-risk pregnancies or the right way to identify and treat hidden depression among black females.

In 2005 Woodard was spending most of her time on the details of the state's proposed Medicaid waiver, which will facilitate enrollment of beneficiaries in "medical home networks" for primary care. "It looks as if health centers will keep their existing advantageous reimbursement rates," she says, "but we are worried about how patients will be enrolled and whether they will be given the appropriate information to make a knowledgeable choice in selecting their provider. In other states it appears that Medicaid recipients don't always know what they're getting into, and then they have to figure a way to get out." The uninsured get a lot of attention, too. Woodard has pursued an innovative partnership with the small firms that are the vast majority of South Carolina's employers and are often unable to provide health care coverage. In coordination with the Small Business Chamber, she is trying to arrange for the businesses to pay most of the health centers' sliding fees for their employees and their families.[26]

Safeguarding the Future

Most of the people who helped start Comp Health are still in the area, their feet planted firmly in the Low Country sand. Gardner continues his stewardship but also looks outward. An athletic man whose hair and beard are beginning to show some gray, his soft-spoken demeanor sometimes belies his widespread influence. His expertise is sought when nearby health center organizations, such as the one on Johns Island outside of Charleston, need help with management. Gardner has been the elected chair of the state primary care association three times and the national health center association once, and he is frequently consulted by federal officials on program policy. His wife, Connie, heads the state vocational and rehabilitation office for Beaufort and Jasper counties. As of 2005 her efforts to retire and travel more with her husband were still meeting with pleas from her bosses to take on new duties.

Elijah Washington served for a time as the first black chief of staff at Beaufort Memorial Hospital, returned to the health center, and retired in 2005, having delivered 10,000 Low Country babies. The local paper cited his dual career as a Baptist minister and his interest in medicine dating back to childhood. "I stood up on a 5-gallon paint can, peeping through a boarded-up window, and saw a baby being born," he explained. "It never left me."[27]

Thaddeous Coleman retired from Comp Health in 2004 after thirty years of service, and reports he is putting his skills to use owning and developing a multipurpose commercial property serving the mostly white, gated resort community of Harbor Island. Emory Campbell moved over to head the Penn Center in 1980 and stayed until 2002, shepherding the historic institution through more reinventions as old problems were solved and new ones presented themselves. He emphasizes that some of the same aspects of Low Country culture he fought to preserve might lead not only to new business ventures but also to more active, healthier lifestyles.

Tom Barnwell went on to campaign for affordable housing and full participation of working-class blacks in the affairs of his native Hilton Head. Retiring in 2005 from the Native Island Business and Community Affairs Association, a group he founded in 1995, he reveled in a roast by his old colleagues. Barnwell has continued to complain that the island's high-priced gated communities discourage cooperation. The fact that they are called "plantations" probably doesn't help. Development has been "economy driven, not community driven," he told an area magazine, and it's taken much too long for people to work together.[28] When I spoke with him in November 2005, he was heading out to attend a family meeting to plan for the long-term use of the land owned by the Barnwells for 150 years. He is also writing a book about the Hilton Head he knew as a boy, before the bridge connected it with the mainland and all the development began. "I don't plan to make myself a vegetable," he told a reporter. "I plan to plant vegetables." And no doubt a few ideas as well.

Barnwell has also become a proselytizer for a study Comp Health has undertaken to help determine risk factors for prostate cancer. South Carolina is seventh among states in the incidence of the disease, which afflicts twice the proportion of blacks as it does whites nationally. The center was singled out to share a $1 million Defense Department grant with the American Health Foundation, the nation's second largest cancer research organization, and then received another $2 million for telecommunications equipment and continued study from the HHS Health Resources and Services Administration. Comp Health screens men for the disease, takes their family histories, and follows their health status and lifestyles periodically through physical exams and interviews, all of which are recorded on videotape and shared with researchers. A lay group meets to keep the activities focused on patients and not just academics.

A prostate cancer survivor himself, Barnwell knows the fear the disease can engender. He says it's "super desperately needed" for local men to participate in the study. Reporting on progress of the research, a local newspaper pointed to the irony that the same health center Barnwell helped to establish in 1970 was now "looking for a cause to the disease that nearly killed him."[29]

Despite many gains and an impressive record of recognition and accomplishment, vigilance is needed to maintain the progress of Low Country blacks, according to Gardner and others. "I don't think we're where we need to be," he says. "The opportunities have increased, but there are still people who think that blacks aren't ready for leadership positions." A black majority on the Beaufort County Council in the 1970s helped Comp Health become a stepping-stone for future leaders, but with the addition of seats reflecting Hilton Head's growth, the balance has tipped back to eight white Republicans and three black Democrats, Gardner says. Moreover, many of the pioneers have retired. Elections director Agnes Garvin believes it's up to young people now. She poses a challenge to them: "If we hadn't done something back then, we wouldn't be in these positions. It's your turn to stand up for yourself."[30]

What does the future hold? Barnwell worries that young people's commitment to equality isn't the same as it once was. "They haven't had the struggle we had," he says. Gardner is more optimistic. "More and more younger people are staying here, or coming back. Look at Louis Dore's sons, joining his law firm. And I'm grooming someone to take over here at Comp Health, just as Tom did with me."

Chapter 5

New York:

Health Care Is a Right

A golden day in Central Park, sun shining on autumn leaves. Enormous medieval pennants hang over the Bethesda Fountain plaza. The rainbow of people includes roller bladers, acrobats, families on outings, dog walkers, and one lone reader sitting yoga style on a glacial rock. The lake is full of boats and the boathouse full of rich tourists sipping $7 Bloody Marys. Those with less money line up for the cafeteria. A hassled maître d' gripes to no one in particular: "How soon do they expect a table when I have to deal with Spike Lee and the *Wall Street Journal*?"

I'm returning to that thick stew of charm and chutzpah, guts and heart, that was my home for fifteen years, my North Star for much longer. I moved to New York in 1960, convinced it was the center of the universe. I came of age here and made the transition from observer to activist, swept up in a deepening commitment to civil rights, my own search for community, and involvement with electoral politics. Things are different now, but on days like this the festival of street life brings some of it back.

The Sixties Happened Here

The sixties happened in many places, but surely they happened here: Hare Krishna dancers, street music, people at card tables hawking not wares but ideas. Depending on which corner of Eighty-sixth Street and Broadway you stopped at, you could sign up to register voters, boycott grapes, or march for peace. And yes, support your local health center. My old neighborhood, the Upper West Side, is home to the William F. Ryan Community Health Center, largest in Manhattan, and now operating sites in the Lower East Side and the midtown Chelsea-Clinton area as well.

The story of the Ryan center, like so many others, is one born of need and opportunity, followed by a struggle to gain independence from the hospital where it was first established. It's also a saga of survival, growth, entrepreneurship, the ups and downs of network development and managed care, wheeling and dealing in the New York political scene, preservation of consumer governance, and commitment to community needs. One health services researcher who interviewed patients from numerous New York centers says: "Ryan is the one place they claim as their own."[1]

The Upper West Side extends from Central Park to the Hudson River, bordered by Fifty-ninth Street on the south and Harlem on the north. Some streets boast turn-of-the-century castles, high-ceilinged apartments with six or seven bedrooms, renovated brownstones, and subsidized housing for lower-middle-income residents. In the sixties, more often than not, each middle-class block had its own pockets of poverty—crowded "old law" tenements and once-proud hotels turned to warehouses for welfare recipients, full of drugs, sickness, and crime.

The residents were just as varied—blacks and old-line WASPs; second-generation Jews and Irish; first-generation Puerto Ricans, Haitians, and Cubans. There were academics, artists, writers, mothers, merchants, and laborers. The checkered condition of the 268,000-person Riverside health district, which encompassed most of the area, brought the infant mortality rate up to nearly 33 deaths per 1,000 live births, compared with citywide and national averages of 26.[2] Some people struggled to give their children a decent life when the smallest mishap could mean eviction, worldly goods in the gutter, a downward slide into disaster. Others just gave up.

But the neighborhood was also home to dozens of clubs and organizations and hundreds of causes, and an incubator for civil rights and community action even before the national awareness of the sixties. Now it was fertile ground for the new programs coming out of Washington.

A Time of Hopefulness

"Think about the idea of a national war on poverty," says Paul Torrens, who came to New York as a young internist just out of the navy and the Harvard School of Public Health. "Or the concept of health care as a right. It was a time of hopefulness, but it wasn't completely naive."

During his stint at Harvard, Torrens had spent some time at the New York City Department of Health. He got to know the commissioner, who recruited him in 1962 to help St. Luke's Hospital reach out to its West Side community. "How does an old-line Episcopalian institution affiliated with Columbia Medical

School and oriented to inpatient care do that? I had three years of support to figure it out," he recalls. "Me and a secretary, an organizational base and a letter-
head. I was happy as a pig in you know what."

The hospital didn't provide much in the way of operating funds, so Torrens
went to Washington and got his first government grant, for control of heart disease through home nursing. Then he got funds to set up a pilot methadone
maintenance program for heroin addicts. Soon there were four locations external to the hospital. "I built a whole unit from soft demonstration money," Torrens says. "It was quite a run. Washington had money but not the community
connections. I'd get on a plane and run into friends who'd ask me how much I
had in my bucket."[3]

Then he heard about the new health center program run out of the Office of
Economic Opportunity (OEO). Torrens knew the area could use such a center.
Catherine Krouser, a black community leader who lived in the giant Douglass
housing projects north of 100th Street, agreed: "This was a booming community and we needed a larger place for primary care. It was more than the health
department could handle. My son's knees are still not right forty years later because he didn't get proper services."[4] Neither did the hospital's episodic outpatient care suffice. Arnaldo Barron, a West Side labor activist, explains: "We
might see a medical resident at the hospital but he didn't know how to take care
of us. The hospitals didn't provide bilingual services for Spanish-speaking people, so they didn't know that an upset or confused person wasn't crazy—just a
human being."[5]

Torrens took a trip to Boston to talk to Jack Geiger and Count Gibson,
who'd started the first centers, and then to Washington to meet with OEO officials. "They told me how to apply and advised me to plug into the political
structure. That meant Congressman William F. Ryan and the city government,
who gave us space in the old health department building on 100th Street,
across from the police station. The hospital said they'd make it work—in for a
dime, in for a dollar."

Some of the trustees didn't get it, Torrens admits. "They wanted to know
why we needed a separate center out in the community when the patients
could just walk another ten blocks to the hospital's main building. These were
people who always held their meetings in the boardroom of a Wall Street law
firm. One woman with that lockjaw accent said she herself hadn't been to the
West Side since she sailed on the *Ile de France*. But it was a remarkable
period—one where we could open up an insular system despite its history."

Torrens drafted a grant application with the participation of several community groups, and put together an advisory board whose members would be

patients of the center, including Krouser and Barron. "Some were reasonably suspicious of our role. Here's this white preppy doctor whose main ally is a black Caribbean nurse. We had a woman from Cuba, a welfare hotel resident, the head of a local tenants' association," he remembers. OEO said yes, and federal health center funding for what was then known as the St. Luke's Neighborhood Health Services Program began in 1967. Based on the model that Geiger, Gibson, and the federal government espoused, the Upper West Side residents who came to the new center received not only comprehensive health care but also patient education, social support, and bilingual services.

"The center was the shaping event of my life," Torrens says. "I was just a do-gooder kid, thirty at the most, running a program with an impact on so many people. It taught me a kind of humility. This wasn't a dress rehearsal; it was life. Early on a cop from across the street offered to take me on a tour of his beat—one of the welfare hotels on Broadway. It looked bad from the outside, and was worse inside—narrow corridors, surly characters, tiny rooms, and locks that didn't work. I'd learned in school about the connection between health care and the rest of people's lives, but it wasn't until then that I understood why the guy we were looking for couldn't come to the center. There was no one to watch his room, and he was sure that what little he had would be stolen. So his congestive heart failure, his leg ulcers, and his diabetes went untreated."

To deal with situations like this, one of the center's highest priorities was training people from the neighborhood to conduct outreach and patient advocacy. Barron remembers the attention paid to respect for the patients: "We wanted to make sure everyone who came in was pleased with the kind of people working at the center. We interviewed job applicants to get a sense of where they were coming from. Sometimes they had a good background but not the sensitivity. Dignity had to come first, then whatever disease the person had."

As important as community employment was, it also left the new center vulnerable to those who wanted to use the patronage for their own purposes. Several years into the process, when the center's budget had grown to $2 million and a lot of jobs were at stake, a Bronx politician attempted a takeover. He was ultimately defeated by Barron, Krouser, and other board members. Krouser says proudly: "When the challengers sent their goons and tried to take us over, it was sheer unladylike behavior that beat them back. They couldn't get a toehold in the health field. Later they went into housing and ended up being accused of fraud."

Self-Determination

In 1969 Torrens left to run a hospital in Hong Kong for the Maryknoll sisters. "By then I was married. My wife had been in the Peace Corps in Colombia and we looked on the offer as a chance for a real adventure together," he explains. But he didn't leave without having recruited the man who had much to do with the center's subsequent growth and development.

Julio (Jay) Bellber, today a hulking ringer for a mature Sean Connery, had come to New York when he was ten. "I was one of the first Puerto Rican kids in a tough Irish area in Washington Heights," he recalls. "I was afraid to go out to the corner store, went six blocks out of my way so I wouldn't have to fight. Then my buddies and I spent a whole winter hacksawing the fence around a neighborhood pool so we could sneak in the next summer. Finally, we were accepted." He moved to the Douglass projects and continued his education, getting thrown out of Catholic school and attending Harren High, which he remembers as "one step above reform school." Bellber says he was terrible in class, bored all the time. "I began working in the evenings as an orderly at the St. Luke's psych ward, and then transferred to medical records. I met an interesting lady who thought I had half a brain."[6]

Rose Tadonio, a short woman who walked with crutches because of a childhood bout with polio, brooked no nonsense. She put Bellber to work organizing the St. Luke's archives and supervising a complex relocation, and then singled him out to set up the health center's medical records. "Rose had taken her department and made it a crackerjack place," Torrens remembers. "Employees wore shirt and tie, and she called them mister. I took her seriously when she recommended Jay." Bellber was intrigued by the center and decided he wanted to work there permanently. "I talked to Rose and Paul and they agreed. I had a lot of ideas about how to organize records, finance, billing, personnel," he recalls. "Everyone else was focused on services."

The hospital bought into the health center board's choice of a neighborhood woman to succeed Torrens as director. But there was little leadership, and things were chaotic, according to Bellber. "I hated community control," he says. "Formally, the board just had advisory powers, but they were actually hiring people who would show up for work without anyone in management expecting them. They could call an ad hoc meeting and turn the place upside down. I told them I would seek their advice, but do my own hiring. And I had to insist on certain policies. Otherwise we had doctors who would keep their records stuffed in a desk drawer." He continues, "Between the director and the board most of the staff turned over. Eventually the community opposed the director and forced her out." Bellber survived, most likely due to a combination of his street credentials, straight talk, and trouble-shooting ability. He says he began to inherit problem areas, and over time became de facto chief of operations.

In 1975 Janice Robinson, a black psychiatric nurse at the center, took over as director. She worked in a kind of triumvirate with Bellber and a white business manager named Barbara Schneider. The years that followed saw board leadership solidified under the direction of Arnold Braithwaite. The son of a noted black poet from Harlem, Braithwaite was a Harvard graduate in chemistry, unusual in the 1940s. His color, civil rights activism, and radical ties had made it difficult to get a job, but during the sixties the liberal Republican administration of Mayor John Lindsay hired him to help run the city's manpower training agency, where Barron also worked. Barron says, "I decided Arnold would be perfect for the health center board. I brought him an application and told him he had to join."

Braithwaite had political smarts, a quiet professional demeanor, and strong commitment to the community. His leadership was important because things were coming to a head with St. Luke's. Krouser recalls that the center's staff had more of a "get more flies with honey" attitude, so the board took the lead in confronting the hospital. "St. Luke's didn't think our board had the experience to run the center. They acted like they were our parents. We were pulling teeth to get respect, let alone coordination of referrals for our patients. Our doctors couldn't follow their patients in the hospital because in those days they weren't all board certified, and the hospital wouldn't send the records back to us." In 1977 the health center and St. Luke's parted ways, with some acrimony. The board, known as the Mid West Side Neighborhood Health Council, became the recipient of federal funds and the center's official governing body with policy-making authority. The following year the center was renamed for Congressman Ryan, its longtime and much-beloved advocate, who had passed away five years earlier.[7]

Then the staff triumvirate began to fall apart. Schneider, who had made significant contributions at the Ryan center and more generally to the nascent organization representing all New York City centers, was diagnosed with terminal cancer. Robinson cared for Schneider's children, and after her death took a job in Washington, D.C., heading the national health center association.

In 1979 Ryan's board selected Bellber as the next director—a choice strongly opposed by the New York regional office of the U.S. Department of Health and Human Services (HHS), which now had first-line responsibility for health centers. Regional staff were concerned about Bellber's lack of academic credentials and wanted Ryan's medical director to move up to head the center. They generally favored health professionals in leadership positions, as evidenced by the fact that New York and New Jersey had a large proportion of hospital-based centers long after most other regions had turned to fully empowered community groups.[8]

Helping Bellber in his quest to stay on as director was a new addition to the Ryan family, Barbra Minch. Described in a *New York Times* profile as a "a firebrand" with a "gingersnap frizz" and "stiletto heels," Minch says she grew up in Brooklyn as a "pink diaper baby," referring to her parents' somewhat left-wing politics and union ties.[9] She attended Boston University, taught in Coney Island, married, had two children, and was soon divorced with little support. "I was on food stamps for a short time," she remembers. In those days Minch got by with the help of a group of women in similar circumstances, celebrating holidays together and creating their own traditions. She taught for a while in East Harlem and then in 1974 came to work for the Upper West Side/Central Harlem school district. "I was heading the local parents council and the superintendent hired me so I wouldn't picket him," she says. It was the heyday of community control, New York's answer to de facto segregation and unequal schools.

Eventually there were cutbacks, and she was laid off. The former chair of the local school board was working as staff to the Ryan board that had just picked Bellber as director, Minch recalls. "Diane Morales introduced me to Jay at Under the Stairs, a West Side restaurant and hangout, and he offered me a job as his assistant." Several years later she was made deputy director, acknowledging the leadership role she came to play in both management and external affairs.

Minch remembers her first whirlwind days at the center: "We had our hands full. The feds rejected our grant application—reams of paper held together with rubber bands, pages cut off in the middle." The application was a mess, and what it revealed was worse. "The regional office asked for a 50 percent reduction in our budget, and then they turned around and used it for bargaining. They said they wouldn't slash our funding if Jay didn't contest the director's job."

She and Bellber appealed to Congressman Charlie Rangel, who had a close relationship with George Lythcott, the head of the HHS Health Services Administration in Washington. Rangel set up a meeting in his Capitol Hill office. "We filed onto the plane to D.C.," Minch remembers. "The health center contingent included our union representatives, Arnold and the board's vice president, Jay and me. An official from the regional office was on the same plane. As we went by he whispered, 'You're gonna lose.'"

In Washington, the group was joined by Lythcott; Ed Martin, who headed the bureau in charge of the health center program; and other congressional staff. Minch says the regional office began a litany of what was wrong at Ryan: the most expensive and underutilized mental health program in the nation, major debts, bank overdrafts. Bellber asked for six months to turn it around. "Charlie walked in from the House floor and asked Lythcott what he was doing to fix the situation," she recalls. "Lythcott determined that Jay would have his six months, submit a reduced budget, and bypass the regional office, reporting directly to Martin."[10]

Too Stupid to Know It Couldn't Be Done

Minch continues: "We started to pull things together, meet with staff, and begin the process of applying for a state license as a freestanding ambulatory care center." She recalls that early on, Bellber fired the medical director, whose productivity was far below par and who had secretly been negotiating his own deal, including budget cuts, with the regional staff.

But the budget did have to be reduced, debts liquidated, and patient services improved—all at the same time. "When I took over the total budget was $3 million, $2 million of which was federal grant," Bellber remembers. "We did a lot of cutting, including contracts for things we could do in-house. We also owed $1 million to Medicaid, $1 million to assorted creditors, and $1 million to St. Luke's, mostly for pensions and administrative expenses. Those were crazy days. Fortunately, the hospital settled for $100,000. Medicaid said they would charge the hospital and the center $50,000 each, but they never sent us a bill. The other creditors settled for 25 cents on the dollar. Once we got straight the center never saw red ink again."

Bellber and Minch attended meeting after meeting with community groups. "We had very little presence out there," Minch recalls. "Few groups knew the center existed. I heard terrible things—patients were ignored, staff were on the phone, the facility was crowded and dirty, there were three-hour waits. It was easy to confuse us with the health department—same problems, same building. At first I knew nothing about health, but there were parallels with education— the need for more resources, judiciously used, and that same professional-paraprofessional split. We met constantly with staff about what we'd heard in the community, from the look of the building to how patients were treated across all levels."

"We attacked everything as it came," Bellber says. "We washed and painted the facility. Doctors who were not busy while patients waited were fired. We set up schedules and demanded that they be followed. We created a service-oriented philosophy." He credits community support for his appointment as permanent director to Minch's "eyes and ears" role. She recalls the turnaround point: "I knew it was getting better when we started hearing positive feedback. We organized a rally at a nearby community center, solidified support, and patient census started going up."

In the midst of all this Bellber was hospitalized for surgery resulting from an old injury. "He wouldn't trust anyone else with our data report to the feds," Minch says. "They had to bring it to his hospital room." Jeff Lattman, an accountant who had pinch-hit at several New York centers, served briefly as acting director. He, Bellber, and Minch forged a close relationship that lasted until Lattman's death years later. "We knew our space at the health department was a big problem," Bellber remembers. "We started planning for a new facility right away. I was learning to focus down the road, not just on what was on top of us. And we were gambling. We built in a margin above the budget so there had to be growth. No growth meant we were losing ground. I was too stupid to know it couldn't be done."

There were major efforts under way to redevelop the Upper West Side, and the Ryan center resolved to be part of them. They identified 35,000 square feet of ground floor space in a new "market rate" apartment building to be constructed at 97th Street and Columbus Avenue, three blocks south of the health department site, and signed a long-term lease. But they still needed a sizable loan for internal construction and renovation—much more difficult to obtain than a mortgage secured by the property. "We applied to Chase Manhattan," Bellber says. "At first they turned us down, but then they began to take an interest. They came over, and we opened up our books." With Lattman's help, the center was able to show that most of the proposed loan could be repaid through Medicaid and other insurance streams. Ryan became the first health center in the country to obtain its own private financing for a major facility.

The center's board played an active role in acquiring the new quarters, with board chair Arnold Braithwaite and Bellber working closely together. "Arnold bought into my vision," Bellber explains. "He brought the board along. Slowly and surely they became more like a corporate board, with administration of the center accountable to them. It took trust for them to accept the leadership of an accountable person." Barron describes the relationship this way: "The board and director need to work together. In the beginning they may think differently but if there's a problem they sit down and work it out. The difference a good board makes—it's like a family. You need a *mami* and a *papi*—one stops and the other says let's go."

Support also came from an unexpected source. After the HHS regional office was overruled in its effort to displace him as director, Bellber says, "I was always in trouble with them, always mouthing off. Then they assigned Rose Forstner as our project officer because no one else would have us. She was the toughest I ever dealt with. We fought like crazy, but we both wanted to do it right, and she became my advocate."

Internal management was further solidified when John L. S. (Mike) Hollo-man, who had been working with Rangel, joined the center as vice president for medical affairs. Holloman's background couldn't have been more suited to a flagship health center, starting with his World War II service as flight surgeon to the Tuskegee Airmen, the renowned black flying unit. In the sixties, he orga-nized and served as the first head of the Medical Committee for Human Rights—the same group that had sent health center founders Geiger and Gibson to Mississippi to care for civil rights workers. In private practice, he broke the color bar at Mt. Sinai Hospital when a famous patient, Sammy Davis Jr., de-manded his presence—only to hand back the hastily approved privileges the next day. In public life, he had served as president of the New York City Health and Hospitals Corporation. Holloman brought prestige and commitment, proudly displaying a plaque with the center's motto, "Health Care Is a Right." But he is remembered most fondly as a mentor and peacemaker. "I could let my guard down with him, show my vulnerability," Bellber recalls. "I'd ask if peo-ple were plotting against me and he'd say yes, they probably were—but some-how he made me feel less paranoid."[11]

In 1988 the Ryan center moved to its new quarters. Conducting a tour for some federal officials from Washington, Holloman pointed to the modern de-sign, inside atrium, and separate waiting rooms for each service. It looked like the physician practices that hospitals had established to capture the new well-off residents of the Upper West Side, but this facility served the uninsured, peo-ple who lived in the projects, even those who had been forced by urban renewal to relocate in other neighborhoods. Puerto Rican staccato and Haitian patois echoed down the halls, spoken by staff as well as patients. Afterward, Holloman heard that some of the feds thought the building was "too nice" for a poor peo-ple's program. He smiled. "What's too nice for people who deserve the best?"[12]

East Side, West Side

"That year was critical for us," Bellber says. "It positioned the center for where it is today." In addition to the new quarters on the Upper West Side, Ryan took over the management of a long-standing health center on the Lower East Side, known as NENA. Many thought it would mean nothing but trouble, but Bellber saw the move as a major opportunity for expansion. "I was like a kid in a candy store," he says. "I wanted to try everything."

NENA had been having fiscal and management problems, and Forstner, the project officer for the Lower East Side center as well as Ryan, began to suspect that utilization reports were falsified. She requested management audits, which found that leadership was all but absent, there were few patients, and revenues were even lower than reported. But NENA's services were desperately needed. The area that had served as a gateway for so many immigrant groups over the years had given way to violence, graffiti-covered walls, and crumbling buildings. Poverty rates were high; drug abuse was a major problem, and the death rate from AIDS, 49 per 100,000 people, was one of the highest in the city.[13] Thus federal officials were reluctant to close the center. Instead they forced the board to accept interim management by contracted consultants, even as they acknowledged that a longer-term solution was required.

NENA's situation concerned neighborhood groups as well. Victor Papa, a former seminarian and radical activist, was director of the Lower East Side Catholic Area Conference, pressing for use of vacant buildings for affordable housing. Papa's group was furious to find that some of NENA's board members were listed as owners of the center's properties and were seeking deals with developers. "A group of little people were playing with a health center built for the poor, trying to enrich themselves, and most local politicians were doing nothing, just letting it fester," he recalls. "We knew NENA was in danger of being closed by the feds. We had to organize the community. We formed a committee— Friends of NENA—and held an enormous public meeting at St. Brigid's Church. Some NENA board members attended. They tried but couldn't defend their actions. Then we went to one of their meetings. They just sat there oozing guilt. We ended up taking over the agenda."

"We went to the attorney general and petitioned the court to remove the board," Papa continues. "They told us to identify a health care entity to act as receiver. We met with some groups who talked about hospitals—totally foreign to our way of thinking, not community based. Then we met with these people from Ryan on the Upper West Side who had been suggested as possible receivers. Jay Bellber—what a bastard—sarcastic, overbearing. And Barbra Minch—a crazy woman, but sensitive to community jargon. She softened him. She developed the personal, he the professional. It seemed like a show they put on." At first Papa saw the Ryan center as a threat to the integrity of the Lower East Side community: "They were less than 10 miles away, but it seemed like the other end of the world. Ryan saw one entity down the road. We saw two and feared one would be ruled by the other. Most of the elected officials from the Lower East Side were also suspicious, and Upper West Side legislators had to intercede." Papa says he got over his fears when he realized that strong leadership was needed, and he came to have great respect for both Bellber and Minch.[14]

NENA's fate was the subject of meetings between state representatives and federal officials flying in from Washington. At issue was whether Ryan would accept the receivership, as well as who would blink first and commit the funds needed to tide the center over. In the end, the feds contributed the bulk of support, with some help from the state, and the court formally named Ryan as NENA's receiver.[15]

Once the decision was made and the dust had settled, a process much like the one Bellber and Minch had been through ensued. Kathy Gruber, who had been in charge of payroll and purchasing at Ryan's Upper West Side center, moved to NENA as assistant manager. She had credibility and solid experience with financial procedures—both sorely needed. But at first she seemed an unlikely choice, having also been the Ryan center's union representative. "Since then I've learned that straight-talking individuals can make a difference whatever side of the labor-management divide they are on," Gruber says.

"In the beginning there was little reason to trust us as caretakers," she recalls. "When we got to NENA we found that services were severely underutilized, and there were revolving door doctors. Several of them turned up on the Medicaid fraud list. The place was a zoo, and even the few patients who came in had been treated terribly. The waiting room was crowded and dirty and a bottleneck for people waiting to get upstairs for services." In its early years NENA had pioneered family-oriented care with teams of doctors and nurse practitioners. Now it had degenerated into a poorly run urgent care center. "No wonder there were deficits," Gruber says. "The previous managers didn't bother to see if the patients were eligible for Medicaid—just put down 'self pay' and charged them $10 a visit. And everyone was in complete denial about AIDS."

"Gradually our hard work paid off, and things began to change," she continues. "The following year the manager was leaving and Jay asked me if I could run NENA. I wanted the job—I was doing everything anyhow. But I needed help. I told Jay he had to be there some of the time. He showed up every Wednesday to mentor me on management and take some of the pressure off. We renovated the facility floor by floor, hired a board-certified medical director with hospital privileges, developed a stable medical staff, reopened dental, increased outreach. After a while it wasn't just day-to-day survival. I could go to community groups and say, 'We're different now.' "[16]

Results were evident in the changing financials. Between the new facility uptown and the improvements at NENA, Ryan's operations doubled. "In July of 1988 our total revenues were $5 million," according to Bellber. "By May 1989 they were $8.5 million and by the end of 1989 $10 million."

Managed Care: The Two-Faced Monster

One more watershed event in 1988 was the formation of CenterCare—a Medicaid managed care plan with a board controlled by Ryan appointees.[17] It seemed a reasonable investment—even necessary. The state had announced plans to move Medicaid beneficiaries into managed care, and several hospital and health center organizations were starting their own plans to capture anticipated revenues and avoid losing patients. But it proved to be the riskiest move of all.

According to Bellber, between 1988 and 1992 CenterCare grew slowly and consistently to 15,000 enrollees and a surplus of more than $15 million. Participation was not yet mandatory for most of the plan's service area, limited to Manhattan. "Then the state said they wanted bigger plans," he says, "and we invested heavily in technology and marketing to become citywide. By 1993 our enrollment was 30,000." But further growth was blocked as scheduled expansion of mandatory participation was postponed in the face of political opposition. For a while, the state stopped all plans from enrolling more Medicaid recipients, even on a voluntary basis.

"In 1994 the bottom fell out," Bellber says. "Our reserves fell below the statutory requirement, and the state came down on us like gangbusters." Ryan's situation was not unique: Across the country, several other health center–based plans largely dependent on Medicaid were stymied by stop-and-go behavior by their respective states. Unlike plans sponsored by some hospitals or private companies, they had no deep pockets to tide them over rough periods. But it was hard for those accustomed to success. "After feeling sorry for myself I sat down with the board and brought in a Wall Street firm to do a prospectus," Bellber recalls. "We knew we needed $10 million to stay alive."

Beth Israel Hospital was ready to make the loan. It was more supportive of services for the poor than many voluntary hospitals, yet competed with the centers for Medicaid patients and stood to gain in the long run if the plan went under. "We insisted on keeping control of the CenterCare board, but the price they extracted was a 'supermajority' on certain issues tied to payback," Bellber says. That meant that the hospital had the final word on operational decisions until the first $5 million was repaid, and on corporate decisions until the full $10 million was paid back.

After the crisis, the loan was repaid and CenterCare's citywide enrollment grew to 80,000, fueled in part by mandatory participation. Then in 1999 there was another rough period. The federal government was pushing Medicaid managed care as a panacea for cost reduction, and facilitating mandatory enrollment at the state level through waivers of regulations. New York State applied for such a waiver. Hospitals that feared revenue cuts were placated with "conversion" money that was used in part for development of new outpatient facilities. "The hospitals wanted their own 'feeder' clinics," Gruber says. "Beth Israel and Bellevue, both located just north of the Lower East Side, opened primary care sites and group practices close to NENA. We complained about the duplication to the hospitals and then to the community planning board but nothing changed. Eventually our managed care enrollment began to grow again." In the long term, she believes, "Health centers are better for patients. Hospital clinics are very visit-specific. They don't see the whole person. We take a holistic approach and look at all of a person's needs. Also people are in and out of Medicaid eligibility. Health centers like Ryan and NENA continue to see patients even when they lose their coverage, but most hospitals do not."

The mid-nineties also brought a restructuring of Ryan's governance, which helped to shelter the health center from managed care fallout and accommodate its increasing size and complexity. The court-ordered receivership had ended, and NENA merged formally with Ryan. A network comprised of the centers and the managed care plan was established, with the majority of its members appointed by the existing health center board.

A New Regime and Emerging Health Problems

Leadership changes were under way as well. Bellber moved up to head the network and CenterCare. The board appointed Minch director of the center, and she carried on the "never say no" tradition in her own way. According to one staffer: "Barbra Minch does not believe in obstacles. She picks away at them until she tears them down." Between 1995 and 2005 the Ryan center's annual budget grew from $26 million to $36 million and the patient population from 25,000 to 34,000.

On the governance side, Arnold Braithwaite, the board chair who had played such a pivotal role in the center's early success, moved to the network level, a position he held until his health failed. He was succeeded by Bobbie Maniece-Harrison, a professor of health education with a nursing background who had been vice chair for ten years. Maniece-Harrison's relationship with Minch is not dissimilar to the symbiosis between Bellber and Braithwaite. "The board had no other thoughts but Barbra for director," Maniece-Harrison remembers. "She was so modest about her salary I had to talk to her at home. She's a wonderful administrator, and she uses her political strength to get some of the state dollars that always flow to the powerful hospital industry."

Maniece-Harrison grew up in an upwardly mobile black family in Alabama—in the same community where Condoleezza Rice spent part of her early childhood. She trained as nurse at Tuskegee Institute and moved to New York in 1964 to study anesthesia. But after working in the operating room, she soon realized she preferred to interact with her patients. Along the way she collected masters' degrees in nursing and community health and a doctorate in health education. "I came to the Upper West Side in 1971," Maniece-Harrison recalls. "One of the first things I heard was that you couldn't live here without being involved." She became active in the Riverside Church and eventually served on the boards of Ryan, the Harlem Young Men's Christian Association, the Greater Harlem Nursing Home, and the New York Coalition of 100 Black Women.

Maniece-Harrison's background helped her and Minch position the Ryan center to deal with a wide range of emerging health problems, from homelessness to the changing face of HIV/AIDS. "The health center movement was started to bring together all types of needed services. Because of that we can influence behavior, and people are less likely to fall through the cracks," the board chair explains. A breast cancer survivor herself, she did her dissertation on the need for early diagnosis of that disease among black women, and she uses her own case as a teaching tool for women who lack support or resources. "I've been able to help so many women because I know how breast cancer threatens your femininity, and makes you reluctant to talk about it," Maniece-Harrison says. Ryan arranges for its patients to receive free mammograms— something many health centers have not been able to do. It sponsors bilingual breast cancer support groups and receives funds raised by the prestigious Revlon Run/Walk for Women—the only health center to do so.

The Ryan center also reorganized the way maternity services are provided, achieving a level of collaboration with St. Luke's that might not have been possible in the early years. "We were offering prenatal care and then referring patients for labor and delivery. It was conservative in terms of costs but less desirable for patient care—you meet a stranger just at the crucial point," Maniece-Harrison explains. "We went from that to having our own obstetricians in the hospital, and soon afterward added eight specialty services on site."[18] Going still further with the rapprochement, early in 2006 Minch reported that the center was actually negotiating to take over the St. Luke's/Roosevelt outpatient clinics.

Ryan's second-tier managers are key to its innovation. Will Murphy, director of outreach and special programs, grew up Irish and gay in and around Boston and got involved in ACT UP, the radical AIDS advocacy group. He sees parallels to the civil rights movement, where activists also organized services that were lacking. He came to Ryan in 1992 to administer prevention and education grants. Over the years, his domain grew to a virtual empire of efforts that promote healthy behavior and get people the care they need. HIV/AIDS services include clinical care, substance abuse prevention, even acupuncture. A project called AirBridge assures ongoing case management, transfer of records and medications for the many HIV/AIDS patients who travel between New York or Connecticut and Puerto Rico. "New York is still an epicenter for HIV," Murphy says. "It's worse than ever. But Ryan has always been ahead of the curve. People like Mike Holloman spotted the epidemic moving from gay white men to people of color. Since I came to the center we're seeing more women and substance abusers as well."

There are also four school-based health centers, services for the homeless in five facilities, and an adolescent outreach and services program known as SHOUT that operates out of a wildly painted mobile van. "Besides general primary care we provide counseling and testing for pregnancy, as well as HIV and other sexually transmitted diseases. We go out looking for runaways, street kids, some in abusive relationships, where we know they hang out. Even the driver is an outreach worker," Murphy explains. "After 9/11 this capacity was called into action almost immediately. Lower Manhattan was a frozen zone, but we could field staff and vans right off the bat. We were out distributing water and meals, filling prescriptions, talking with the elderly, and ferrying shell-shocked people to emergency rooms."

Murphy's latest project: He's found a way to relate to people over the age of fifty who might be at risk for HIV. "It's an emerging population and we need to do more with them," he says. "We offer a monthly seminar on a general health issue—vision, breast cancer, mental health. Then we end with a little *novela*, or soap opera, about two people who meet, get together and wonder what to do about sex. The focus is on characters and intimacy, not disease. Our patients keep coming back to find out what happened since the last cliffhanger. To our surprise, they're also eager to talk about their own experiences."[19]

The Least of Our Brothers

When he's speechifying, Congressman Charlie Rangel is fond of asking a biblical question: "What have you done for the least of our brothers?" Then he lets you know that health centers are up there among those who have answers. The people at Ryan, the center in his district, spend a great deal of time and effort assuring a continuum of services for the uninsured—roughly 30 percent of the patients they see.

Visit them on any given day and many of the senior administrative staff, up to and including the director, are involved in coverage problems. Uninsured people are frequently refused treatment elsewhere and end up at Ryan. The center's existing patients need specialty and hospital care, and for those without insurance it's often like pulling teeth.

Maria Lugo handles most of these referrals. She's a lifer—an Upper West Side resident for all of her forty years, a Ryan patient herself as a child, and an employee dating back to a summer youth program when she was fifteen. "Then during college I needed a part-time job, and they hired me as a cashier," she says. "When I graduated I came to work here full time." Today Lugo oversees patient services—a twenty-six-person unit responsible for registration, internal and external appointments, and patient accounts, which includes shepherding Medicaid applications through the complex approval process.

While her duties are technically demanding, Lugo also views them personally: "My job is to advocate. If you help someone once, you're stuck. They bring their problems to me, and I help them navigate the system. They feel terrible enough asking for a handout. To be made to feel helpless compounds the problem. So they come here because they feel a connection with us. When I was a kid people would say they were going to the clinic—every one knew they meant Ryan. A hospital—that could be anywhere."

Lugo has had her own experience dealing with impersonal and self-defeating bureaucracies—her family's displacement from their home by urban renewal, and a widowed mother who fell through the cracks because she didn't fit into any of the categories that would have made her eligible for health insurance. "I would go with her to apply, and they would call out a list of names, with no effort to pronounce them correctly," she says. "You're not human to them."

She would like to do away with the restrictions that make coverage such a patchwork affair—income (of every 400 people who come in to the Ryan center, 250 earn too much to qualify) and eligibility for children but often not their parents. Another favorite target: the huge cost of having all the forms go back and forth, and the extra time spent on annual recertification. "Sickness is a big business," Lugo says. "My money would go to universal coverage, but a lot of people don't see that it's an important investment until they get sick. Is it cheaper to pay now or later—that message has not gotten across." She understands that part of the reason for opposition to expanded insurance is people not wanting to pay more taxes, but thinks bias against minorities is also to blame.[20]

In fact, for a state with a progressive reputation, New York has a surprisingly high proportion of uninsured—16.7 percent of the nonelderly population, just slightly under the national average of 17.8 percent. It's the highest proportion of any state in the Northeast or Mid-Atlantic region. The city abounds with new immigrants, many of whom are undocumented, and service industry jobs that don't offer coverage. And while Medicaid payments are by far the nation's most generous, averaging a total of $7,800 per enrollee annually, rates for private physicians are among the lowest, severely restricting availability of care.[21]

"Whatever change comes must be bottom up," Lugo believes. "And it should reinforce that people must be treated with respect and dignity." Until then, she says, "I must set an example so I get mad, curse, yes—in my office by myself."

David and Goliath

Where do Ryan and other health centers fit in New York's complex panoply of providers, given hospitals' claims that they serve the vast majority of the city's uninsured and low-income people?

Judy Wessler runs a watchdog group called the Commission on the Public's Health System. Started in 1991 to fight privatization of the city's public hospitals, its agenda has broadened to address access issues—keeping hospitals honest and getting resources to providers who serve low-income and uninsured New Yorkers. "We do research, policy analysis, organizing, assistance to community groups, and butt kicking—my favorite because there are a lot of butts that need kicking, and I don't mind doing it," Wessler says.

"People try to dismiss the role of health centers in New York because there are other providers of care for low-income people," she continues. "But the centers are critical—there's such a lack of priority for preventive and primary care, so much goes to fancy equipment, high-tech care, barring the door to those who can't pay. We don't have enough health centers or enough resources for their services. I'd like to expand their capacity and fund a richer package—paying for diagnostic procedures like MRIs, as well as specialty care, to deal with referral problems."

Half of those living in New York City are either uninsured (1.8 million) or on Medicaid and other public insurance (2 million). Wessler estimates that of roughly 11.5 million ambulatory care visits by this population, maybe 1.5 million are to health centers and another 1.5 million to entities that look like health centers in terms of access and at least some of the same social and support services. Private physicians also play a role with Medicaid recipients, but in terms of sheer numbers, the hospitals do provide the bulk of low-income outpatient care. However, there are major differences between the hospitals' and health centers' mission and focus.[22] For ambulatory care provided by voluntary hospitals citywide, the "bad debt and free care burden" is 11 percent of total costs, while in the city hospital system, established to provide care to all who need it, it is 24 percent. In Manhattan, for voluntary hospitals the figure is also 11 percent, and in the city hospital system, 18 percent.[23] An exact comparison with health centers is not available, but the Ryan center reports that 30 percent of its patients lack coverage; 40 percent of its revenues is from grants and other contributions for care of the uninsured and special facilitating services not covered by insurance, while 60 percent is from payments by patients and insurance plans.[24]

When it comes to influence, the health centers and access advocates play David to the hospitals' Goliath. The Greater New York Hospital Association (GNYHA), headed by transplanted midwesterner Ken Raske, has formed an alliance of unprecedented power with Local 1199 of the Service Employees International Union (SEIU), led by Dennis Rivera. Hundreds of thousands of hospital jobs are at stake.

Raske defends the hospitals' role in providing free care, citing individual institutions that serve larger-than-average numbers of uninsured. It is true that some could do more, he says, but changing priorities is difficult in the face of managed care pressures and federal funding reductions. He believes that at bottom, the indigent can get care in New York. "Maybe they go through some portals to find it, but look at the operation to separate the Siamese twins in the Bronx. The family was uninsured, and it cost millions." On the other hand, Wessler says that the hospitals' obligations to provide charity care are poorly monitored and probably underrealized. "There's a firm suing hospitals all over the country, including some in New York, for not meeting their free care requirements."

Raske also disputes claims that he doesn't work with health centers: "We lift a lot of water for them—I disagree that there isn't cooperation." Among common interests, he cites fighting Medicaid cuts, increasing eligibility for Family Health Plus (state coverage for parents building on the federally supported State Child Health Insurance Program), and moving the agenda on health insurance more generally. His proposal—to expand employer-based coverage by assessing those who don't provide insurance—is logical: "Now we fund hospital care through a tax on premiums," he explains, "so those who do provide coverage get a double whammy. This would be probusiness in the sense of spreading the burden." But so far, as in many states, fiscal conditions haven't been conducive to passage.[25]

The real muscle—and the results—of the GNYHA/SEIU lobbying efforts can be seen in huge sums of new money flowing directly and all but exclusively to hospitals. First was the $1.25 billion in conversion funds that came with federal approval of the Medicaid managed care waiver discussed earlier. New York was not the only state to provide a sweetener for providers and patient advocates leery of managed care, but most others in similar circumstances used the money to expand public insurance. Commented the *Village Voice*: "So overt were the project's politics that part of the deal was struck in November 1996, when Rivera brought Governor George Pataki over to talk to [then vice president] Gore at the Al Smith dinner—the Catholic Church's annual political event."[26]

Health centers were told that to share in the conversion funds, they had to seek money from hospitals in their areas—not practical in view of the competitive climate. After extensive lobbying, the state finally gave them a pittance of $4 million to be shared by a total of fifty organizations. A subsequent evaluation of how the hospitals spent their funds by the Commission on the Public's Health System found that, for the most part, they supported routine expenses and established new facilities in areas already served by health centers or in otherwise well-supplied suburbs. Many hospitals did not submit required reports to the state, and Wessler had to file a Freedom of Information request for the data that did exist.[27]

The hospitals and the union repeated their coup in 2002 when Empire, the state's not-for-profit Blue Cross plan, was acquired by a for-profit organization. States typically share in the proceeds of such transactions, in recognition of the tax and other benefits of not-for-profit status the plan received in past years. Most have used the "windfall" to establish charitable foundations that expand access and support community interventions. In New York, Governor Pataki struck a deal with GNYHA and SEIU, which had opposed the Empire sale, to channel most of the funds directly to hospitals for wage increases on the principle that employees might be adversely affected.[28] Again Ryan fought hard for a share, and health centers got minor concessions. Minch says it helps that they are one of the few centers to be unionized and maintain good relations with union chief Rivera.

Many hailed Pataki as a genius. Months later, running hard for reelection as a Republican in a state with a Democratic majority, he was endorsed by Rivera's union and won. The sum of money involved with Empire's sale increased from an estimated $1 billion when the deal was struck, to over $2 billion at the time of the initial public offering, and to a whopping $4.8 billion in 2005 when the new for-profit plan was acquired by its parent company, WellPoint.[29]

"Extraordinary," New York assemblyman Dick Gottfried says of the Empire deal. "Just like the managed care conversion money. It is a good case study of the continuing struggle between health centers and hospitals." The state assembly is the larger house of New York's bicameral legislature, and Gottfried has chaired its powerful health committee since 1987. He says an important part of his work is trying to steer additional money to the health centers and strengthen them financially. "Before I took over as chair of the health committee," he explains, "I had a rudimentary knowledge of health centers, mainly from Ryan, which was not far from my district. Then I began to learn more about where they fit into the system. They fill what would otherwise be a major void."

He sees the centers not as a substitute for but as complementary to the expanded insurance coverage he has fought for. "Poor people who have Medicaid are a lot better off than if they were uninsured, but even they have problems getting quality health care," Gottfried explains. "There is widespread unavailability of primary care practitioners in low income areas and reluctance of doctors to accept Medicaid. It's somewhat better with Medicaid managed care, but people are still using emergency rooms and outpatient departments to a large extent. With health centers, care is more accessible and affordable, the patient is more likely to see the same experienced practitioner twice in a row, as opposed to rotating residents, and the community control elements help keep services in line with people's needs. The model is eminently successful for low-income people, but I think it would be attractive even for those with higher incomes and excellent health coverage."

"Advocates for health centers and poor people generally believe that hospitals suck up an enormous amount of health care funding, they are big and politically powerful, they compete for the same insured patients as centers in some neighborhoods, and they aren't as good at delivering primary care," he continues. "To a large extent, I agree. I consider myself a significant friend and helper of hospitals that serve a large proportion of the uninsured, but it's clear that the centers do a better job of primary care, and they certainly don't get a fair share of the money. We could use twice as many health centers."

A Third Site

Gottfried thought enough of Ryan as the preeminent Manhattan center that when his district was shifted south, he sought the center out to help bring services to his new area, where a report by the city health planning agency had documented a severe lack of primary care resources. Different from either the checkerboard demographics of the Upper West Side or the grueling poverty of the Lower East Side, the neighborhood includes Midtown, Chelsea, and Clinton (more colorfully known as Hell's Kitchen). There are industrial properties, more tenements than brownstones, public housing, and subsidized apartments for artists and actors.

"In the early nineties when I first started the work that resulted in the Ryan/Chelsea-Clinton site, we brought in a group of people—health policy experts, advocates, the local hospitals—to talk about what to do," Gottfried recalls. "But from the start it was clear to me that the solution was to get someone to put a health center in the area. Before we knew it we were cajoling Ryan to do it. It was a combination of urging them on and then paving the way. I helped with the state license and certificate of need, and the bonds to raise money. An astonishing and prolonged pulling of teeth was needed to get all the pieces in place. And then there was the community's concern about the color of the bricks on the building's facade."[30]

Bellber also remembers the endless meetings, time, effort, and seed money contributed by the Ryan network to get the project off the ground. The latest addition to the Ryan family opened in 2001 in a new building with brick similar to other structures in the area, but with teal trim that matches the center's other sites. New York senator Hillary Rodham Clinton has visited several times, amused that the neighborhood and the center's time-honored name is the same as her daughter's.

George Lowe, the site's deputy director, lives in and knows the community. A New Yorker by birth, he worked as a military health administrator in Washington, D.C., and then moved back to New York, where he headed the HIV/AIDS program at St. Clare's hospital. "I was part of the movement to get the program established when this neighborhood was hit so hard hit by AIDS," he recalls. "Helen Hayes helped because St. Clare's was known as the theater hospital, and Mother Teresa drew attention to the problem."

Eventually Lowe took over the hospital's other ambulatory care services as well. When he moved to the Ryan/Chelsea-Clinton center, he saw it as an opportunity for real service integration. "An AIDS patient could be sitting next to someone who is commercially insured, a Medicaid recipient, or a homeless person," he says. "It takes away the stigma." In addition to medical, dental, and mental health care, services include a small wellness center with massage, acupuncture, yoga, and meditation. "The neighborhood people love it," he says. The homeless are more integrated into the community as well, according to Lowe. "The Salvation Army and another street-to-home program called Common Ground help them get Medicaid, decent clothes, and good shelters. When the shelters needed TB tests for all their residents on a two-day turnaround, we got them done."

From a financial and a clinical point of view, the area's demographics pose both opportunities and challenges. "This is a transient area," Lowe explains. "The rents are high for new buildings and the apartments small." There are more elderly people and fewer families with young children. For the center's patient population, that translates into 10 percent children, compared with 40 percent at the average center, and fewer people with Medicaid, the best payer. There's substantial commercial HMO coverage, and more uninsured than at Ryan's other sites. And there are a lot of seniors with Medicare, Lowe says: "Show people, what they call 'one-hit wonders' from the sixties, and people who moved to the area to care for family members with AIDS and stayed on. With an older population the health problems are more complex."[31]

Trouble in Paradise

By 2004 Ryan's purview was nearly boroughwide. Not only the largest center in Manhattan, it was recognized nationally for leadership and innovation. But more changes were coming.

The organizational structure—health centers, on the one hand, the HMO and network operations, on the other—exposed fault lines that were several years in the making. Other large centers throughout the country have had similar problems when entrepreneurial leaders move up to operate at a higher level. There are inherent conflicts between centers, driven by their unique mission to serve the underserved, and an organization that must compete with moneymakers and profit through its own investments. The two are not mutually exclusive—the centers certainly enjoy power and money and the HMO/network is not oblivious to mission, but the nature of what they do can lead to diverging interests.

In the case of Ryan, Bellber wanted to maximize managed care enrollment for CenterCare—understandable given the history of having to go hat in hand and ask for a bailout. He insisted that the health centers not participate in other managed care plans, which was not consistent with the position taken by the majority of center-controlled plans across the country and conflicted with the centers' interests.[32] "We were losing patients who enroll in other plans because of it," according to center board chair Bobbie Maniece-Harrison.

Another issue involved use of profits or surplus. Bellber said the surplus didn't belong at the center level, where funds are subject to federal rules and may be used to offset grants in future years. He also didn't want the funds to lay idle. His vision was to create a revenue stream and build an endowment for the centers. The network invested in a software company, technology services, and venture capital, in some cases with national and state health center organizations. The Chelsea-Clinton site is one example he uses for the kind of payoff he envisioned. The center leaders, who had helped capitalize the HMO, would have liked some of the profits for immediate needs. A greater difference between them and the network was that they took a more conservative position on the appropriate level of investment risk. "Our first responsibility is to protect the center's assets," Maniece-Harrison says.

For many years Minch had been Bellber's "eyes and ears," protecting his back and, as others have noted, moderating while he pushed. Now that they were in separate organizations the differences in personality and temperament seemed to come to the fore, not just with Minch but the other center leaders as well. In addition, the whole group of respected advisers who might have softened the differences—Braithwaite, Holloman, Lattman, Forstner—had passed away.

The result was increasing separation between the health centers and the HMO/network. At the same time, circumstances were ripe for the sale of CenterCare. Enrollment had stabilized, there was less opportunity for growth, rates were being cut back, and the proceeds could be invested elsewhere. In June 2005 the center-based HMO was sold to Fidelis, a not-for-profit Catholic plan whose executives said they were pleased at the community service aspects of the acquisition.[33] The Ryan network was dissolved, and the profits of the sale were shared, with one-third going to a charitable foundation directed by the centers and two-thirds to a foundation headed by Bellber. CenterCare and the Ryan network used to share an office on West Fifty-seventh Street in midtown Manhattan—a building where the hospital association and other HMOs are quartered. They had a startlingly beautiful view of the New York skyline—tens of thousands of skyscraper lights against a night sky. While Bellber hasn't lost his Puerto Rican accent or street-fighter demeanor, he puts it this way: "Dealing up there you have a different view of the forest. You see the horizon, not the woods."

Always the Street Life

Down below, it's always the street life. It's a powerful memory for Paul Torrens, now professor of health services and former department head at the UCLA School of Public Health. "You'd go outside and there was this direct exchange with the community. I'd take the kids for a walk in their stroller, and I'd always see patients and board members. Bill Ryan would go up and down Broadway, thanking people."

Today high rises line Columbus Avenue—formerly the domain of cut-rate stores and problem buildings—and they are filled with higher-income residents. Half of the Ryan center's patients now come from north of 110th Street—Washington Heights, home to many new immigrants, and the multiproblem Central Harlem area, which still has some of the city's worst health statistics.[34]

According to Catherine Krouser, the Upper West Side has gotten "boozhie," and the pockets of poverty are smaller. But, she says, "I still love this neighborhood." She and Arnaldo Barron remain patients at Ryan. Her mobility is limited, and the center has helped her acquire a motorized scooter so she can continue to keep an eye on what's happening in the streets. Barron says: "I've always had my own doctor here. He speaks to me in Spanish. When a vein broke in my retina they sent me to one of the best specialists in the city." The center is large enough to require a security department, headed by a veteran of community policing recruited from the precinct across from its original site. The retired West Side Irish cop fusses like a mother hen over patients and staff alike.

The other sites have their street life, too. At NENA, there's a demonstration over how much of the center's old disputed property will continue to be used as a community garden and how much will go for a planned collaboration with Henry Street Settlement to build assisted living for the neighborhood residents. The important thing is that there are two noble purposes, and no developers in the equation, according to one observer.[35]

At Chelsea-Clinton, an art exhibit hung on the long lobby's open walls is just opening. Some of the featured artists are patients. Wine and cheese are being served, and the crowd spills out the door and onto Tenth Avenue.

Krouser's favorite event is the annual holiday party, always held at one of the sites. In an age of glitz, it's still informal—ethnic food, lots of drink, and high spirits. If you look around, you can see the vestiges of all those families that inhabited Ryan over the years—Barbra Minch and her friends creating new traditions, Jan Robinson caring for her dying colleague's kids, the *mami* and *papi* Barron likes to talk about, multiple generations of employees, and the old-timers who come back every year.

Chapter 6

The Rio Grande Valley of Texas:

Steps from the Third World

Down where the Rio Grande splits southernmost Texas from Mexico, rich soil and a subtropical climate have always attracted year-round crops and the poor people who work them. In recent decades hundreds of thousands more have been drawn to the region by some 250 maquiladoras—large U.S.-owned manufacturing enterprises perched on the international border to take advantage of a cheap labor force and greatly reduced import taxes.[1] To the workers on the Mexican side, just up from the abject poverty of their country's mountain regions, the average hourly rate was attractive at $1 plus change, and it's been rising in some places.[2] So they crowd into unincorporated *colonias* without education, health, or sanitation services, and try to do more than just survive. Dooryards are painted in bright colors, and some feature small gardens. But there is barely enough to eat, and white plastic bags from the communal dump blow across scruffy fields like some strange kind of tumbleweed. The single source of water is full of rats, raw sewage, and industrial waste. Now, in addition to poverty, the Rio Grande Valley breeds toxic pollution.

On the U.S. side of the border, being poor is different. The average worker makes four times as much as his or her Mexican counterpart—the mean hourly wage in the Brownsville-Harlingen Metropolitan Statistical Area is roughly $7 for agriculture and $8–9 for industrial machine workers.[3] The problem is not eating too little but eating the wrong things; not lack of transportation but lack of exercise. Big Macs and French fries have replaced subsistence living, children are overweight, and diabetes is rampant.[4] Primary care is available for some, but the local health center's waiting rooms are full to bursting. The proportion of people without health insurance is greater in Texas than in any other state.[5] When uninsured people need specialty services like chemotherapy or in-patient care, they still drive 480 miles roundtrip to the nearest public teaching hospital in Galveston.[6] Housing, schools, sanitation, and other services are much better than in the past. But history and proximity are constant reminders that this part of Texas is only steps from the Third World.

History Turned on Its Head

Forty years ago, conditions in towns like Brownsville and Harlingen, and especially out in the countryside, were much more like those in neighboring Mexico. Hardship was a way of life, in part because of isolation. The counties in the triangle bounded on the east by the Gulf of Mexico and the west by the Rio Grande were cut off from the rest of Texas by the King Ranch and other agricultural giants.

Perhaps more important, a tradition of violence and exploitation haunted the area. In the Rio Grande Valley, the history most U.S. schoolchildren learn is turned on its head. The Alamo is no heroic stand, and the ultimate victory over Mexico in 1848 is a tragedy of major proportions. All of the land south of Corpus Christi was ceded to the U.S., and the formerly Mexican Hispanic families who owned property for generations were suddenly subject to a new regime. Things got really bad around the turn of the century as land values soared, agriculture replaced ranching, and Anglo farmers sought to remove the Hispanics from their land with the help of zealous Texas Rangers. A Hispanic rebellion centered on the counties in the Valley was put down with much bloodshed.[7] Domingo Gonzalez, a local activist, says many a family has tales of forebears who were scalped by the Rangers.[8]

This period was followed by a different type of violence. Historian David Montejano writes that racism came to the fore after 1920 as Hispanics worked as sharecroppers on Anglo farms and the Valley's population of agricultural workers swelled each growing season with Mexican immigrants, crossing a very permeable border that artificially split families and friends. In places where the population was mixed, schools, living arrangements, and political organizations were segregated.[9] The area also served as a staging ground for those who continued their journey north to pick crops in the midwestern states, or up the East and West coasts. Many lived in squalid labor camps or the U.S. version of service-poor *colonias*.

Historically, Hispanics comprised almost 90 percent of permanent residents in Cameron County, where Brownsville and Harlingen are located, and still do.[10] Yet according to longtime activists, as late as the sixties nearly all state, county, and municipal officers in the southernmost part of the Valley

were Anglos. Those in power, with a few exceptions, were conditioned to accept the harsh conditions faced by the area's indigenous people.[11]

In 1960 the infant mortality rate in Cameron County was 35.5 per 1,000 live
births and in rural Willacy County, 45.1, compared with 29.1 for the state of
Texas and 26.0 for the U.S.[12] These proportions persisted in the overwhelmingly Hispanic area despite the general tendency of Hispanic infants to be born
healthy.[13] Many babies failed to thrive or died before their first birthday of uncontrolled diarrhea, conditions related to malnutrition and widespread pollution of water supplies. Natives called it *agua peligrosa*. In addition, a variety of
skin diseases, including leprosy, were common.[14] Basic health services were
all but absent for those who couldn't pay. Stories like this one abounded: "A
woman we knew went to a local hospital in the late stage of labor. She was on
the delivery table when they asked her for $5,000. She got dressed, took a bus
to the border, walked across the bridge to the city of Matamoros, and went from
doctor to doctor searching for help. She had an arm and a leg hanging out by the
time she found someone to deliver her baby."[15]

How Community-Based Health Care Came to the Valley

In 1968 an "unholy" alliance of young Volunteers in Service to America (VISTA)
workers, local activists, and Catholic Charities hatched the idea for a health
center aimed at the Rio Grande Valley's migrant and seasonal farmworkers. Dan
Hawkins, a red-haired Irishman straight out of Boston College, says he joined
VISTA—a domestic version of the Peace Corps that was part of the War on
Poverty—to do good and avoid the draft. His dual motives were not uncommon
for the time. "I had majored in Spanish so they sent me to South Texas," he remembers. "Along with several other volunteers, I was placed in the Cameron
County community action agency. They asked us to go out and see what people
needed most. Health care was high on nearly everyone's list, and so was clean
water."[16]

Domingo Gonzalez was working on clean water and health care issues in
the *colonias* upstream along the Old Chisholm Trail. "There were a lot of little
groups in the Valley counties," he remembers. "We came together as the Organizaciones Unidas, and we stole Dan Hawkins to help us. He and two other
VISTAs became friends with the meanest, ugliest crowd in the towns, and got
them involved. There was also a reformed redneck who became Mexicanized,
and a guy who played the harp in bars as an organizing tactic."

This loose confederation targeted the federal migrant health program—
consisting at the time of funds disbursed by county health departments to local
providers at $50 to $60 a visit. "It wasn't working," Gonzalez says. "By midyear

when the migrants came back from the north the money was gone. We decided we needed that money for a clinic that would meet people's ongoing needs, and we sought an alliance with the Catholic diocese." The Catholic Church was a force for liberalism in those days, he explains. "They didn't interfere, and they were more supportive than the labor groups here, who had their own pro-development agenda and focused only on jobs."

Many of the same people involved in health care were also fighting for voting rights and backing Hispanic candidates for office. "It was the Hispanic version of the civil rights movement," Hawkins says. "And, like black activism, it was growing more radical. The national Hispanic advocacy group, La Raza Unida, was the closest thing to a separatist political power this country has ever seen."

At this crucial point, near the end of 1969, the federal government withdrew its support for the VISTA volunteers in Cameron County. Hawkins recalls that legislation sponsored by Congresswoman Edith Green of Oregon had given state and local officials greater authority over community action agencies. In this case, the VISTAs, with their support of voting rights and agenda of controlling federal health funds, were seen as a threat. "It was actually a boon to us," Gonzalez says. The Catholic Charities extension program took up the salaries of some of the VISTAs, and Hawkins eventually became planning director for the community action agency. "Dan went to D.C. on begging tours for the Valley. And Billy Sandlin of the federal migrant health program agreed to come down to see us."

The upshot, according to Hawkins, was a compromise that allowed Cameron County to keep its migrant health grant of $350,000 and awarded another $350,000 to a new organization known as Su Clinica Familiar—Your Family Clinic. Su Clinica was one of the first "reformed" migrant programs at the Department of Health, Education and Welfare (HEW), adhering to community health center principles of comprehensive services and consumer involvement. "At the last minute the feds balked at handing over money to a community group," Hawkins says. "In short order Catholic Charities agreed to serve as a conduit. It was a faith-based program in the best sense. The diocese provided strong support behind the scenes, but they only had one person on the center's governing board, and they deferred to decisions made by the community representatives."

"We wanted to target Brownsville first, because it had the largest concentration of Hispanics," Hawkins explains, "but politics wouldn't allow it. There was a city-county clinic in Brownsville, staffed sporadically by volunteer doctors who didn't see the need for anything else." So Su Clinica opened its doors in a tiny Harlingen storefront on May 5, 1971. It was Cinco de Mayo, the date widely celebrated as Mexican Independence Day. "Our first patient was a diabetic whose leg was so gangrenous it had to be amputated the next day," Hawkins remembers. "He said he didn't seek help sooner because he already owed $3,000 for his daughter's care, and in his family, the kids came first."

An Anglo known as the "Connecticut Yankee" was an unlikely choice to head the new program, but the community pushed for Hawkins to become director. Gonzalez was a board member. Paula Gomez, a sixth-generation resident of Brownsville, came to work at Su Clinica as a researcher and statistician. She had studied journalism and biology in college and vacillated between work at a local hospital and the nearby resorts on South Padre Island. "They were both plastic," she says. "I wanted something else, and I got it."

At the health center, Gomez's organizational skills soon got her promoted to clinic manager. "Early on there was this little guy, maybe two months, whose mother brought him in from La Paloma. He was in terrible distress, dehydrated from uncontrolled diarrhea. He stopped breathing, and we gave him oxygen. The doctor ran for his car. 'Keep up the oxygen while I drive to the hospital,' he said to me. But it was too late. We were in the elevator going up to the pediatric ward when the baby died in my arms." Gomez continues: "I learned a lot that day about how to keep going when you think you've failed. It made me want to learn about public health, and so much more. It was the beginning of this thing that eats you up and doesn't let you go."

Beg, Borrow, or Steal

Staff at the new center knew they were just scratching the surface, and they set out to patch together the resources they needed. At first there was only one doctor, William Heusel, a general practitioner in his late forties. A devout Mennonite from Nebraska, Heusel had gone to medical school late and committed to one year of service in a place of great need when he had completed ten years of private practice. When Su Clinica opened a small satellite in Raymondville, twenty miles north of Harlingen, he single-handedly staffed both clinics for a year. Before leaving, Heusel helped recruit a young general practitioner and fellow Mennonite, David Enz. At the same time, the center recruited Paul Todd, also a general practitioner and one of the earliest assignees of a new federal program known as the National Health Service Corps (NHSC).[17]

In 1972 Sister Angela Murdaugh, a no-nonsense Third Order Franciscan nun involved with migrant outreach, became the first of her order assigned to Texas. Trained at Columbia University, she was an early pioneer of nurse midwifery. "At first Dan Hawkins didn't know what to do with me," Sister Angela says. "He thought maybe I should go for my Ph.D. But he learned that I could open a maternity service and run it. There wasn't room at the Harlingen clinic so I went to Raymondville to set up a freestanding birthing center in May. We delivered our first baby there in July." Sister Angela's birthing center was a resounding success, at first among Hispanic women who couldn't afford hospital deliveries and were used to native midwives, or *parteras*. "Later, it became so popular that Anglo women starting using it," she recalls.[18]

When another nun from Sister Angela's order came to visit, Hawkins convinced her to stay on and use her training to establish a home health agency under the center's umbrella. A second group of nuns, Dominican sisters, arrived courtesy of the archbishop of Boston, Humberto Medeiros, who had previously been bishop of Brownsville. The center had gotten a foundation grant for a mobile clinic, Hawkins recalls. "A board member and I flew to Cleveland to pick up a used but fully equipped medical van. Driving back, we only broke down once. Once back in Harlingen the van, staffed by one of the Dominicans, visited five outlying communities on a regular schedule. Our doctors provided backup via a CB radio, giving orders for care and deciding who should be transported to the main center."

Stan and Nivia Fisch were New York student activists when they met and married in 1970. They worked and trained in the Bronx at Montefiore Hospital's social medicine program and the Martin Luther King health center, and were involved in the Lincoln Hospital Collective—all hotbeds of radicalism. They ran across Fitzhugh Mullan, who described the world of medical politics in his book *White Coat, Clenched Fist* and went on to head the NHSC, and Ed Martin, who later headed the HEW bureau responsible for community health centers.

Like Paul Todd, the Fisches had volunteered for the NHSC and selected Su Clinica as their practice location, arriving in 1973. Having dealt with the concentrated urban poverty of the South Bronx, they were not shocked at conditions in the Valley, although it took a while for them to find their niche. The need for doctors was so severe that Hawkins persuaded Stan, a board certified pediatrician, to see adult patients. But he was concerned that Nivia, a family nurse practitioner, wouldn't be busy enough. "They didn't know what an NP was, and they wanted to pay me as a licensed practical nurse," she recalls. "I played every role, from medical records supervisor to clinic manager. And as a liberal woman, I wasn't accepted in the community right away." Then Sister Angela suggested training in midwifery at the University of Mississippi. Nivia returned to start a new career delivering babies in a second birthing center at Su Clinica's Harlingen clinic, now in larger quarters.

Eventually, Stan's pediatric training served him well, as he developed a close relationship with Valley Baptist Hospital. Enz had applied for and gotten admitting privileges, well ahead of physicians at most health centers. Stan followed suit. Not only was he accepted on staff, but he also began to consult with the hospital on professional matters. "When I got here the private medical community was schizophrenic about the health center," he says. "They didn't like government programs in general, but they were supportive in the specific. They could see that we were competent, and they understood the need for care. We were fortunate that Valley Baptist accepted our patients and didn't pressure us to get them out, the way we heard other area hospitals did."

As time went on, the staff grew and the center moved to still larger quarters in Harlingen. "It seemed like a barn of a place, with dirt floors and concrete walls, when we first bought it," Stan Fisch recalls. "But when it was renovated each of us had his own office for the first time." Additional space was needed because Su Clinica was now receiving community health center as well as migrant funds, and seeing nonmigrant patients. The expansion was discussed at great length because of fears that migrants would be squeezed out, according to Fisch. For more than a year, the center put off implementing new federal requirements to collect Medicare and Medicaid reimbursements and to charge patients who could pay on a sliding fee scale. "It didn't seem worth it because so few were eligible, and we were suspicious that the fee scale would be a barrier," Fisch says. "It turned out not to be the case."[19]

Beyond the center's walls the political picture began to change, according to Gonzalez. "It happened in just a few years, like day and night, after 150 years of Anglos consolidating their power. By the mid-seventies there wasn't a major institution without Hispanic representation." David Montejano confirms this transformation occurring all over southern Texas. He says that segregation all but ended, and elected officials began to reflect the makeup of the population not only because of the civil rights movement of the sixties but also because of the rise of a skilled Hispanic labor force in the wake of World War II and the Korean War.[20]

In the Valley, Gonzalez explains, "the process we went through in organizing and setting up the health center helped serve as a catalyst. The most important product was empowerment. We were now positioned to do something about the public health hazards that caused disease." Hawkins adds: "One of our most significant advances was actually a water project we spearheaded to deal with the constant gastrointestinal problems we were seeing. At the board's request our sponsor, Organizaciones Unidas, got a federal grant and built a potable water and sewer system for the outlying *colonias* along the U.S. side of the Rio Grande. Over 2,500 families were served, and disease was substantially reduced—a perfect example of a center that went beyond medical care to improve a community's health."

Shifting Focus

In 1977, with Su Clinica ready for additional growth, Dan Hawkins responded to some feelers put out by the administration of newly elected president Jimmy Carter. "I had been asked to help organize a visit to South Texas by a committee charged with oversight of the national health insurance proposal," he recalls. "I met Karen Davis, who had been tapped for a key position under HEW secretary Joe Califano. I saw her again when I went up to D.C. to testify before Congress on behalf of health centers. She took my hand to shake it and said, 'Come work for me.' I had so much going on in the Valley—growing the center, and maybe running for office—but that was an offer I couldn't refuse."

The man Hawkins favored as his successor said no. He didn't want to deal with the whipsaw politics that had always characterized Su Clinica's board but were kept under wraps as long as the founding director was around. The job was filled by Frank Gonzalez, who wasn't nearly as popular as Hawkins was with community activists or health providers. "I thought Frank's motives were questionable," Stan Fisch says. "He went to a private practice for his own medical care—something none of us would do." Fisch became the center's first medical director, and tried to push for application to the Joint Commission on Accreditation of Hospitals and less reliance on the NHSC, which had its own competing personnel system. But, he says, "Frank was leery of doctors, and he kept me away from the board." Eventually, Fisch resigned the position and in 1982 left to start his own practice. In 1992 he was elected chief of staff at Valley Baptist, holding that position for three years.

Sister Angela left to start her own freestanding birthing center in 1983. After a sabbatical in Washington, D.C., where she learned lobbying and served as president of the national nurse-midwifery association, she says she was eager to try her hand at independent practice. Nivia Fisch followed suit the same year, "for personal and political reasons." For one thing, she recalls, the center director wouldn't negotiate with her as director of midwifery. She affiliated with the local ob-gyn group, whose members knew her work because they had provided backup at the birthing center. At first she focused on prenatal care, with only limited privileges at Valley Baptist. That changed when her husband became chief of staff. He wrote the protocols that let her and other certified nurse midwives manage labor and perform hospital deliveries.

Frank Gonzalez consolidated his power and built a substantial endowment for the center. "To his credit, he kept the clinic going, hired good people," Stan Fisch says. "They finally got accreditation and recruited a more stable group of doctors." Paula Gomez remained as clinic director, administrative aide, and personnel director, working with the community and helping secure their support. Even with most of its old leaders gone, Su Clinica continued as an important and growing source of care. Turnover was not infrequent among health centers generally. But while the Fisches tired of the politics and grantsmanship they associated with a government program, they stayed on in the area, which was uncommon for "carpetbaggers" from the North.

Meanwhile, things were finally moving in Brownsville, at the southernmost end of the Valley, thanks to Mayor Ruben Edelstein. According to Hawkins, Edelstein guarded his power closely and made sure that the likes of a VISTA volunteer from Connecticut didn't gain a toehold in his city. But he was also driven by a powerful commitment to the poor. Mel Huff, a reporter for the *Brownsville Herald*, gives partial credit to Edelstein's family background. "They came here as peddlers, and sold kerosene stoves and furniture on credit," she explains. "A cold snap came, and they'd go around to see if people were getting enough heat. A hurricane threatened, and they got a rope to help evacuate their neighbors near the shore."[21] When Edelstein became mayor in 1975, one of the first issues he tackled was public transportation—then nonexistent in and around Brownsville. "The people on the outskirts couldn't get to work," Edelstein recalls. "We established a bus system that still operates today—one of the few in this area. We also started the only emergency medical system south of Corpus Christi," he says proudly. "As an elected official you have to take responsibility. If you don't want it, you shouldn't run for office."

Health care for low-income people was troublesome, Edelstein remembers, because the city-county volunteer physician services were so inadequate. To make matters worse, the poor population in the Valley was burgeoning due to an economic crisis in Mexico. "The people were not getting enough attention, and the doctors were trying to send those with Medicaid for private services. Some needed it, and some didn't. The uninsured were flooding the emergency rooms, and the hospitals complained that they weren't equipped to handle it." Edelstein had the city assume full responsibility for the volunteer facility and set out to secure federal health center funding. "To get a grant we had to have an ongoing operation and the endorsement of the county medical society. A friend of mine—a former mayor and retiring physician—helped us meet the eligibility requirements. Another friend, Bob Strauss, who was chairman of the Democratic National Committee, interceded." The Brownsville Community Health Clinic got its first federal grant and two NHSC physicians in 1977.[22]

Just after he joined the federal government, Hawkins was asked by health center bureau director Ed Martin what he thought of the arrangement. "I understood the need in Brownsville all too well," he says. "It wasn't the program I wanted to start there, but I knew the political forces behind it would get something going. At least they had a community board, albeit one that shared power with the city administration. I thought they should go for it."

In 1984 the Brownsville center needed a new director. Paula Gomez, looking for a promotion and a move closer to home to care for her ailing mother, interviewed for the position. But she faced formidable opposition. She explains that Edelstein, while no longer mayor, still wielded power and feared her ties to Hawkins. "He thought I would merge the clinic with Su Clinica." Then there was the fact that in south Texas, traditional attitudes about women die hard. "The board gave me the old story about how a single woman without kids didn't need as much money, and they offered me 20 percent less than the outgoing director had made," she recalls. "I decided to hang tough. Then I got a call from Sal Meir, the migrant health director in the federal regional office, telling me to take the job. He wasn't someone I could easily ignore."

Headless Babies and a Stop on the Underground Railway

Now Brownsville was poised to inherit the mantle of activism that Su Clinica had started with over a decade earlier. Gomez had her hands full establishing personnel procedures and hiring and training new employees. The Brownsville center remained in the city facility but spun off as a nonprofit community group, allowing more flexibility in administration and additional revenue opportunities.[23] But she also couldn't say no to people in need. "We went from five to sixteen doctors in two years," she recalls. Her activist penchant was shared by medical director David Smith, an NHSC pediatrician assigned directly from his training at the prestigious Children's Hospital of Pennsylvania. "David was appalled at the lack of equipment and infrastructure, and the hardships 'his' kids had to endure. He wanted to call the media right away," Gomez remembers. "It seemed like one battle after another." Getting the Brownsville doctors privileges and their patients admitted to the two local hospitals was a struggle, unlike the arrangement Su Clinica had with Valley Baptist. Events began to break, and health issues got a lot of publicity when Smith ran for the local school board and won.

Health in the Valley was about to get more attention, this time on the national news. "Three anencephalic babies were born in a thirty-six-hour period," Gomez recalls. "The national average for conditions as severe as those we saw was five per year." The infants had only a vestigial brain, most of the skull was missing, and if they were not stillborn they died within hours. "We went through the gamut of reasons," she explains. "The suspected cause was an environmental insult during pregnancy, possibly benzene from the maquiladoras. People were living a mile to a mile and a half downwind of the industrial park. We called the Centers for Disease Control but decided they were moving too slowly and we would do our own thing. The One Border foundation, formed by our center and spun off as a separate entity, teamed up with the University of Texas Medical Branch (UTMB) at Galveston to sample water and air."

"Certain facts were undisputed—the anencephalic babies; gestation time was affected; calves had been born without brains; 600 fighting cocks were dead," Gomez says. "We did our studies, but it was a political year on both sides of the border. Mexico held back their data, and their epidemiologist disappeared. They called and told us not to come to Matamoros. Domingo Gonzalez, who was working with us as an environmental activist, thought we were on a kind of blacklist. We had only data from the U.S. side." A few weeks later there was a suspicious accident, Gomez continues. "We never proved it was done on purpose, but Domingo was crowded off the road and slammed into a telephone pole. His leg and foot were crushed, and he was left to die. He survived but spent nine months in a nursing home recovering his mobility."

Due to the lack of information from the Mexican side of the border and alleged intimidation of the scientists involved, as of 2005 no article had been published in a scholarly journal. Gomez believes that UTMB turned the information over to a Johns Hopkins University researcher with too-close ties to the maquiladora industries. The One Border foundation had to sue to get the data back. But Smith, who had gone on to become the state health commissioner, helped get the story to ABC News, and they blew the issue wide open. As a result, Gomez says, there is a national registry for neural tube defects—the overall diagnostic category that includes anencephaly.

What's also important is that people like Gomez and Gonzalez haven't forgotten the human cost of pollution in the Valley. Gonzalez dwells less on his own injuries than on what's happened to the area he loved as a child. "The Rio Grande is no longer a river but merely a trickle from Laredo down to its mouth at the Gulf of Mexico," he says. "When we were growing up it was clear, and you could see giant alligator garfish jumping, like prehistoric monsters. They survived the Spanish, the Mexicans, all manner of natural toxins. Now we've lost 200 freshwater species, and if you see just a little needlefish you're lucky." Part of the problem, he claims, is lack of monitoring. "Population has increased five times over on the U.S. side and ten times in Matamoros in the last forty years, and yet there's the same money to monitor industrial effluents. It's the state's job, but they announce the date and time they're going to check two weeks in advance so the factories can clean up—temporarily."

Gomez is concerned about the emotional impact of the infant deaths. "One of the anencephalic babies was ours," she explains. "A couple of months after it was stillborn the mother, a little nineteen-year-old girl, came to us crying uncontrollably. The hospital had told her the infant would get a decent burial. When she went back to get her things an uncaring nurse said, 'You must be the owner of that brainless baby we're keeping in a jar.' I helped her find $500 for the pauper's grave she was entitled to, and we got the county judge to find a funeral home so she could put her child to rest."

Another crisis Gomez describes involved an influx of 2,000 Nicaraguans on the outskirts of Brownsville, just on the U.S. side on the border. "Someone left a very sick child in need of hospitalization on our doorstep," she recalls. "We sent a medical team to their camp. It was cold and damp, and more people were getting sick. We helped them set up tents and began transporting people in our own cars from the camp to temporary medical headquarters we had set up in a nearby gym." Then, she says, "an immigration lawyer called to warn that the FBI was following us. Even when people are already in the U.S., if you take them any further it's a crime. We didn't stop. It was our version of the underground railway." The Brownsville center's connections with community leaders continued to be important. "Bishop Fitzpatrick said he would bail me out of jail if necessary," Gomez remembers. Ultimately, immigration advocates and the National Migrant Referral Project helped the Nicaraguans get asylum.

Where Insurance Is Rarer Than Hen's Teeth

Paula Gomez goes on with the Brownsville story: "After David Smith left and there was less publicity, the hospitals ousted us again. Our NHSC doctors were considered transient, and our patients were not welcome. We'd get phone calls saying, 'Your people ruin the aesthetics of our hospital. They're cluttering up our halls.' Sometimes to buy time we would send our patients south to hospitals in Matamoros, where conditions were primitive but they had generous hearts." Another ploy: "If we needed to hospitalize a patient in Brownsville we'd keep her in our clinic, start an IV, and wait until 5 P.M. when there were fewer administrative staff at the hospital and we'd have a better chance of sneaking her in." There was some improvement when the federal government began to require states to cover medical emergencies for those who would otherwise be eligible for Medicaid, regardless of immigration status. But it took a class action suit supported by the health centers' national association before Texas implemented the new law in 1989.

Eventually the hospitals changed their staffing bylaws and admission policies. Is it better now? "Ah, it's nearly the same," Gomez says ruefully. "Our docs are *allowed* to hold positions in the medical structure, but the hospitals don't really try to help us. They find more subtle ways of keeping our patients out. And for specialty services, our working poor patients travel 480 miles to Galveston and back for subsidized care and still pay thousands of dollars for some procedures." Another problem is that private doctors "dump" additional uninsured patients on the health center. These patients show up with little notes, according to Gomez: "Report to Brownsville Community Health Center—this person cannot afford my services." Other health centers face the same situation, but in Brownsville the volume is overwhelming—over 70 percent of patients lacked insurance in 2005, and the federal grant, used primarily to subsidize the uninsured, is 43 percent of the center's total revenue. At Su Clinica in Harlingen, only twenty-five miles to the north, the proportion of patients lacking insurance is 50 percent—still higher than the national health center average of 40 percent but less extreme.[24] In part this may be because there are more new immigrants in the southern part of the county who have not qualified for public insurance.

In some ways the business focus of the health care industry has made things worse. Emily Alpert came to Brownsville as operations director in 1998 after working in the early nineties with David Smith at Parkland Hospital, Dallas's large public facility. She explains, "Health care has become more of a commodity since one of Brownsville's two hospitals, Valley Regional, was taken over by Columbia-HCA. In addition, this part of country is notorious for large employers with part time workers and large numbers of domestic and agricultural workers with no health benefits."[25]

In 2004 Texas had the country's highest proportion of uninsured people—27.3 percent of the nonelderly population, compared to a national average of 17.8 percent and 9.8 percent for Minnesota, the state with the lowest proportion. The Texas Medicaid program, the safety net for the uninsured, had one of the nation's least generous eligibility levels, covering only 11 percent of all low-income adults.[26] In the view of political pundit Molly Ivins, Texas has a habit of "taxing low and serving little."[27]

A series of articles in the *Brownsville Herald* personalizes the problems of uninsured patients. One is a former nurse with severe lupus, bankrupt from extensive prior surgery, who cannot find a specialist to treat her. Another, a home health worker who discovered a lump in her breast in April, had to wait until September for a mammogram and biopsy and until December for surgery while she looked for providers who would see her at a reduced rate.[28] According to Alpert, the health center staff are fighting every day to get care for people like this. "It's so frustrating. You're the rat at the end of a maze," she says. "There's no comprehensive system. We've got to have secondary and tertiary care for everyone."

Gomez says there are problems getting even a small amount of local money to subsidize specialty care for the uninsured. "Local government does very little in the way of health services," she explains. "The county does immunizations and rodent control. They do prenatal care but no deliveries; TB tests on Tuesdays and diabetes tests on Thursdays. The city deals with stray animals and inspects restaurants." Staff from Brownsville and the other health centers in the Valley are trying to get the three-county area designated a state health district, which would mean allocation of tax dollars for indigent care.

Previous planning efforts have left confusion about the number of people who would need the new services—the health centers and local hospitals use different methods of measuring volume. The health centers have been sharing their information with the dean of a local university to develop overall planning assumptions. Discussions with county officials are ongoing, but as of 2005 there was no increase in state resources for indigent care.

A Tale of Two Health Centers

Despite persistent problems, much has changed in the Valley since the first health center was established. In 2005 there were four such organizations, and a total of forty-nine throughout the state.[29] Su Clinica, the area's oldest federally funded center, was also the largest, serving 27,000 people at its main site and five satellite clinics.[30] Brownsville, whose history as a city-county clinic goes back even farther, served 20,000 at its main site, two satellites, and two school-based clinics. The population in Cameron County increased from 151,000 in 1960 to 368,000 in 2004, but it was still 86 percent Hispanic and 33 percent poor.[31] The two centers share high proportions of Hispanic and low-income users, similar health problems, and careful attention to physician recruitment and chronic disease management, with a special focus on diabetes, which is twice as prevalent in the Valley as it is nationally. Each organization is at the cutting edge of safety net care in different ways.

In October 2002 Su Clinica moved to a new two-story, 62,000-square-foot facility built for them and leased back by Valley Baptist Hospital. It's near the hospital campus and expansive by health center standards, with a porte cochere, manicured grounds, and large parking lot. Inside, it's clear that patient flow was a factor in the design. The decor is tasteful and professional. The building is only the physical evidence of a groundbreaking arrangement with the hospital and the University of Texas Health Science Center at San Antonio, making Su Clinica a principal regional ambulatory care training site for seventy-six third- and fourth-year medical students and a new internal medicine residency program.

Elena Marin took over as Su Clinica's executive director in 1995, when Frank Gonzalez moved from that position to board chair. She's a Brownsville native whose own odyssey includes a local college, pharmacy school in Houston, an M.D. at Boston University, and a pediatrics residency at Duke. She came to the health center with the NHSC in 1986, and served seven years as medical director. Marin is proud of Su Clinica's record in increasing availability of important preventive services to people with diabetes and reducing the proportion with high-risk levels of hyperglycemia.

Another source of pride is the new medical teaching program. "Physician recruitment has always been an issue for us," Marin explains. "When I arrived most of the NHSC doctors were here for two years and then gone. Not many came from this area or spoke Spanish. There were benefits to us but not continuity of care for the patients." Later, when there were fewer NHSC placements available, Su Clinica had to learn to recruit and retain its own professional staff. It was a major challenge and a stressful time for the center. "During my tenure as executive director," she continues, "retention of physicians became much more stable as we began to look at how to keep our doctors in the Valley."

"Bringing students to our center was one way to address physician shortages, but Su Clinica also wanted to be involved in education," Marin says. "We have a lot to teach the students about our families and how best to care for them." In addition, Su Clinica's role as an academic center enhances its visibility and credibility. According to Marin, all Su Clinica physicians have faculty appointments—a major bone of contention in other health center teaching arrangements. "They contribute in a meaningful way to the education of future doctors and help reduce physician shortages in South Texas."[32]

Early in 2006 change also came to the Su Clinica governing board, which hadn't always had an easy relationship with the center management. Some members had held their positions for many years, in contradiction to the board's bylaws. The board members were ousted and the center placed in receivership by a local court until a new board could be constituted.[33] Stan Fisch was pleased with what he called an end to cronyism. Other observers would not go that far, but they agreed that while events did not reflect negatively on the management of the center, periodic rotation of the board members was desirable and consistent with community representation.[34]

Achievements of the Brownsville center include a cutting-edge improvement of its own—automation of medical records, which is strongly recommended by practice management experts but thus far a rarity among health centers. The center attacks the epidemic of obesity and diabetes in the Valley not only through its regular medical services but also by going directly to young people in the schools. The school sites, known as Campus Care centers, provided health education, mental health services, and a full range of primary care services to over 3,000 students of the city's elementary, middle, and high schools. Alix Flores, who directs the school-based program, reports that obesity is a huge concern. "When I grew up here my mother cooked every day—fruit, vegetables, rice, beans," he says. "Everyone played outside. Now you can feed a whole family fast food on $10 a day. Kids lie on the couch, play computer games, and watch TV, and everyone has a car." Exercise and diet are major components of a new effort aimed at schoolchildren.

The main health center is a one-story building of white-painted cinder block. Inside, it's crowded but cheerful, with migrant art posters on the walls. A new facility is being built but meanwhile the waiting room is packed— mothers with babies and older couples. An alternative school for pregnant teenagers across the street sends some of its clients to work at the center. The neighborhood consists mostly of small but neat homes lining a street that is literally the last exit to the U.S. Miss the turn and you cross the Rio Grande into Mexico.

And crossing into Mexico is something Brownsville staffers do routinely. "When you grow up here you understand that the border is just a small bridge with little men dressed in blue overseeing traffic between one side and another. You don't think anything of eating lunch, or shopping, or commuting to work in another country," Gomez explains. "We don't only share the business end, but water and air as well. And we share disease. We worry about outbreaks of cholera, typhus, typhoid and dengue fever. And if TB isn't treated properly in Mexico, there will be drug-resistant TB here."

So the Brownsville health center sponsors work on the other side, not with federal grant dollars but through the One Border foundation and a program known as Mano a Mano. They targeted some brand new *colonias*, where people who have recently migrated from the interior of Mexico live in lean-tos outside the municipal service area. It's like the earliest days of health centers in the U.S., when the purview was much broader than health. "We organize donations of food, clothing, shoes, supplies," Gomez says. She shows me the school they erected. Once the building was available the city of Matamoras began sending teachers, and soon there were 300 students. Clearly, the operating principle is "if you build it, they will come." The One Border foundation also put up a small dispensary, staffed part-time by a physician, a nursing nun, and a social worker. "We're hoping that the medical school will rotate their students through," Gomez says. They also use *promotoras*, or community outreach workers, who are helping count rat bites and sightings. Next on the list: cleaning up the drainage ditch where the rats breed, and making sure it stays clean.

Keeping the Flame Alive

Over time, the Valley's health centers spawned an unusually vigorous and diverse group of pioneers who left an indelible mark on the community. Even with their New York backgrounds—he's kept the tightly wound demeanor; she looks like a shorter version of J.Lo—Stan and Nivia Fisch are confirmed Valley residents, raising a family here and involved in politics and civic life. Early in 2006 Nivia Fisch is still delivering babies with the same obstetrics group. Stan Fisch's pediatric practice on the outskirts of Harlingen is thriving, and he is serving on the board of Valley Baptist, helping plan for the academic partnership with Su Clinica. "Back in 1998 Elena Marin was giving a report on the health center's activities," he recalls. "The hospital board applauded spontaneously, and then voted their support for the new building. I thought wow— how different from thirty years ago. Health centers are important models of care. They've trained a lot of people, and they've moved from the periphery to the center of the local health care system."

Sister Angela is still operating the Holy Family birthing center near Weslaco, now offering the only out-of-hospital deliveries in the Valley. A cluster of board-and-batten buildings are painted bright yellow, surrounded by playgrounds and gardens full of hibiscus and bougainvillea. There's an office, an education room with donated computers, living quarters for staff, and several identical birthing suites—a family room, furnished linen closet, linoleum floors, lots of toys and books, a back room with a double bed, bassinet, and changing table. "Everything's in the same place—it's easier for staff," she says. Women and kids are everywhere. The mothers stay for twelve hours after birth, often with their other children.

Staffed by five nurses and four nurse midwives, the birthing center is delivering 200 babies a year. While there are backup arrangements for emergencies, Sister Angela reports that only 5 of the 200 births required hospitalization. She still delivers breech births and twins without Caesarian section—"a lost art," she says. Holy Family exists mainly on charity contributions plus a unique charge and barter system. If possible, patients use Medicaid or private insurance, or pay $1,500 for prenatal care and delivery. Those eligible only for emergency Medicaid, which provides much more limited coverage, have two options: pay an additional $500, or pay $100 plus the family provides 100 hours of work at the center. And, Sister Angela says, "These are the hardest working people I know. Anyone who says different is crazy."

Modern medical practice may make it difficult for the fiercely independent nurse midwife to continue going it completely alone. Gomez and Alpert from the Brownsville health center helped her with the complex paperwork required for new federal privacy provisions under the Health Insurance Portability and Accountability Act, and they were hoping she would consider collaborating with a private primary care group. Sister Angela explains that she wants something stable, not subject to government whims or red tape. "You can work hard to build something and in the blink of an eye it's gone," she says. "I'm not antigovernment—I'm a dyed-in-the-wool Democrat, but government is too rigid, and I don't want to spend my time writing grants." Programs that cut services for the neediest when faced with shrinking resources are her pet peeve.

Domingo Gonzalez is still an environmental activist, involved in water issues in the Valley. After we talk, he is about to depart for the World Water Forum—an international meeting where he plans to push for the restoration of rivers like the Rio Grande by cleaning up the creeks and smaller streams that feed them, and recycling water supplies instead of building more dams. Gonzalez also works against World Bank support for corporate takeovers of local water supplies, which he says have produced poor results in the Valley.

Dan Hawkins worked for several years at HEW and then joined the National Association of Community Health Centers. Harking back to his early success finding support for Su Clinica, he became the health centers' lead advocate in Washington. But his years in the Valley also left him with a rare understanding of how the small demonstration program evolved into a major actor on the health care scene: "We made our place in forgotten places, among marginalized people," he says. "They are the ones we're indebted to. No one paid much attention until we were an integral part of the community."

Now the question is how to step up to leadership in the larger system and still keep the old dedication and commitment alive. My last night in the area, Paula Gomez and I are having a dinner of Gulf fish on nearby South Padre Island, overlooking the water. She talks about the nine Americorps volunteers at her center—the heirs to the VISTA program that once sent Hawkins and others to the Valley. She was recently invited to Florida to speak to them and other

Americorps volunteers working at health centers across the country. Some were jaded and cynical, she says. "I heard that they had spoken of their bosses at the centers as degenerate hippies."

"They asked me what I would leave them with. I told them how they took me back to my early days at Su Clinica—how I too found myself working with a group of left-over hippies who wanted to save the world. They were all brilliant but it was like a MASH unit—every day a call to action, seeing patients in dire need and then staying up until 3 A.M. to prepare for a board meeting, taking po-litical and personal risks. I told them about the baby who died in my arms; that every time I pass the clinic waiting room and see the faces of people who need us, I think of that baby who died for no reason. Sheer determination—and some naïveté—helped us to be part of a larger dream."

She had some ideas about what the volunteers could take away from their health center experience: "In ten years, when you are briefcase-carrying execu-tives, remember when you are shifting papers and dancing around an issue that once there was poverty and hopelessness, and your efforts changed the face of health care for disenfranchised and marginalized people. And no matter how smart you are, remember that the people you are serving still know more than you."

The final prescription from her own experience: "You need the fire to with-stand waves of helplessness and despair. You need not to know 'no.'"

Chapter 7

The Health Center Legacy

Paula Gomez's advice to the young volunteers is a perfect introduction to this final chapter. We are constantly admonished to learn from history, but as I have traveled around the country I've also seen a jarring disconnect between the rich, emotional legacy of health centers and their need to compete in a modern marketplace as sophisticated providers. Daily life is a constant struggle with the bottom line, and conference schedules are crowded with management techniques, financing strategies, and sales pitches.

And yet the health centers' remarkable story not only enhances their worth in today's world, it also inspires an ongoing commitment to their survival. Like all things of great value, the centers are enriched by their provenance—the telling and retelling of how they came to be created and who has touched and changed them along the way.

Bridging the Gap between History and Reality

What can we learn from the history of health centers and their heroes, especially the up-close-and-personal stories in this book? Despite widely varying circumstances, there are more commonalities than differences, and some important lessons for the future.

Origins

Some centers started with an outside "instigator"—Jack Geiger in the Mississippi Delta and Columbia Point, Paul Torrens in New York, and Dan Hawkins in Texas. These three had a vision and supportive institutions to help make it come true. For others—the Boston centers originally organized by the city government—the instigator, Jim Hooley, was a native son. The centers in South Carolina and Jackson, Mississippi, were started by local activists Tom Barnwell and Aaron Shirley, respectively, who had a history of challenging the establishment on their home turf. While the outsiders were no less dedicated than the natives, they had less at stake in their daily lives and had to face issues of trust and sometimes race, being white in minority communities.

Leadership

Scratch some of the most sophisticated leaders and you find simpler beginnings—people not originally groomed for leadership. Jay Bellber in New York says he was "a loser in school" and didn't start to develop management skills until a supervisor "thought I had half a brain" and took him in hand. Neither he nor Tom Barnwell was a college graduate. Tris Blake at Boston's South End was a high school dropout. Like others in his neighborhood, Jim Hunt took a job in city government right out of high school, and finished college on what he calls the "ten year plan." L. C. Dorsey started as a sharecropper, and Barbra Minch was a single mother, on food stamps for a while. People in Boston talk about how the health center movement "raised them up," paying for training or yielding on-the-job experience they could never get in school. While some federal officials fought the ascendancy of "uncredentialed" leaders, others, like Richard Boone of the Office of Economic Opportunity (OEO), emphasized the importance of street smarts and peer recognition.

Interestingly, the first generation of health center leaders I interviewed were all men—perhaps in keeping with prevailing custom of the early sixties. Some even said it was their wives who got them involved, then stepped back and let them assume the leadership role. In many cases, the second- or third-generation leaders of the same centers were women who came into their own but still agonized over their salary requirements and sometimes had to accept lower pay than men in the same positions.

Where these innovative leaders go when they leave their centers and how they manage the transition is another issue. In two places I visited—New York and Jackson, Mississippi—inherent conflicts came to the fore when successful center directors moved up to the network level. Other early leaders left the health center world for government, advocacy, hospital management, or academia. Current directors of centers in Texas, South Carolina, and Boston are content to grow their operations within the same structure. All of these executives are nearing retirement age, although only Roland Gardner made a point of noting that he is grooming a successor.

Governance

Community governance has been essential to the program's survival, but no one ever said it was easy. Rogue boards in some places have fired excellent center directors or even manipulated resources for personal gain, as they did on New York's Lower East Side before that center was placed in receivership. Successful organizations thought hard and long about who was on the board, what information the board members received, and how they related to center management. Early on, Bellber had to take a step back from a board whose members wanted to make management and personnel decisions themselves, rather than overseeing the executive's actions. As board chair, Arnold Braithwaite became a partner in Bellber's aspirations for the center, and the director came to favor the "two strong people" approach—one on each side of the board/management divide.

In Texas, Hawkins had to refuse resignations from board members who thought they didn't know enough about health. "That's not your job," he told them. "Your job is to tell us what you need."[1] Most of the neighborhood centers in Boston had less trouble getting people to serve on their boards—they were the same people who picketed city hall for services and took hammer, nails, and paint to early facilities. Geiger points to the danger in accepting recognized community leaders who may come with their own agendas, unprepared to listen to people who need the center's services. Although the National Association of Community Health Centers regularly provides training for local board members, more research is needed to demonstrate the impact of consumer governance and identify factors that contribute to its success.

External Influence

In South Carolina, Mississippi, and Texas, the centers not only drew strength from the civil rights movement, they irrevocably altered the white power structure that controlled the economic and environmental determinants of disease. Notably, the center in South Carolina "changed the color of government." It's no coincidence that these centers served rural areas with smaller-scale government entities and dire, highly visible problems of a Third World nature.

The problems of urban neighborhoods—drugs, crime, homelessness, and hopelessness—were harder to deal with and influence more difficult to come by. In the sixties, southern governors were expected to be racist, but big city mayors and institutions thought to be on the side of the poor also opposed OEO programs. Don Sykes, a former community action agency director, observes that citizen participation was not natural to the Democratic power base of public unions and middle-class professionals. "Social workers fought community action agencies, teachers fought alternative schools, and black physicians in private practice fought the health centers," he explains.[2] It's often said that one of the major contributions of the War on Poverty was as a launching pad for the first generation of minority political leaders, but change was a long time coming.

The establishment of national and state health center associations contributed to external influence, perhaps most successfully in Boston, where the Massachusetts League of Community Health Centers was able to defuse racial tension, secure significant state funding, and document economic impact. Mississippi, South Carolina, and Texas all have strong associations. New York, with its multilayered political structure and fractious health centers, has been more problematic. Individuals seem to matter more. Barbra Minch cultivates state and national officials the way she does community activists. "It's in her blood," said a *New York Times* profile.[3]

Health System Challenges

Relationships with hospitals continue to be an issue in both major cities I visited. The institutions have overwhelming political power in New York, as evidenced by the blatant allocation of profits from the sale of the state's Blue Cross conversion benefits to hospital employees. But there may be signs of softening as Ryan and its old sponsor, St. Luke's Hospital (now St. Luke's/Roosevelt), collaborate around specialty services and, more recently, negotiate the health center's assumption of responsibility for the hospital's outpatient clinics. In Boston, there's a patina of noblesse oblige—real in some cases and only skin deep in others. One group of hospitals was described as "circling vultures" over the short-lived bankruptcy of the East Boston center. In both cities, the situation has been complicated by competition around managed care and the need for center-based plans to seek temporary bailouts from the same institutions they compete with. Managed care was far less pervasive in other sites,[4] although it was expected to be implemented in Mississippi, where both the Jackson-Hinds center and the Medical Mall had been adversely affected by state plans that did not materialize, and South Carolina appeared to be moving toward locking patients in to ambulatory care "medical homes."

The Cutting Edge of Excellence

In addition to the macrolevel studies of quality and effectiveness cited in chapter 1, nearly every health center I visited has something important to offer mainstream medicine. In Massachusetts, the East Boston center operates a demonstration in all-inclusive care for the frail elderly that may be a model for keeping seniors of all incomes out of nursing homes. In New York, Will Murphy at the Ryan center has developed new and successful methods of reaching adolescents and older adults at risk of sexually transmitted diseases. In South Carolina, Roland Gardner is using telemedicine to research prostate cancer among blacks. In Mississippi, Aaron Shirley spearheaded the Jackson Medical Mall, an innovative partnership with foundations, health department programs, and the University of Mississippi Medical School. And in Texas, the Brownsville center features cross-border initiatives, and Su Clinica Familiar has become a major ambulatory care training site for medical students and residents.

Values

Many of the health center leaders I spoke with are deeply religious. They emphasize that their faith is entirely compatible with the participation and ownership of their diverse communities and not at all consistent with requiring staff to adhere to a particular sect. Imagine applying a religious test to a center where Catholic nuns and Jewish medical students work side by side with Baptist deacons. "I consider my work to be the deepest manifestation of my beliefs," East Boston's Jack Cradock explains. "It's respectful and inclusive; not exclusionary."

Those who are not formally observant are value-driven, and all are concerned about passing on those values. There was a surprisingly unanimous view, especially among minorities who had to work hardest to get where they are, that values are lacking today. "We learned it at the dinner table," says Helen Barnes of Mississippi. "My wife and I worked late into the night to improve health care and education, and we passed that on to our kids," Shirley recalls. "Our people wanted jobs, not welfare," echoes from John Hatch in Mississippi, Gardner in South Carolina, and many others.

I started my research with a question about how the early leaders found the courage to stand up to certain danger. It's related to this issue of values, whether the answer involves simply doing a job the way it should be done, a debt to those who had laid down their lives, a quest for social justice, or, as civil rights activist Fannie Lou Hamer said, just feeling "sick and tired of being sick and tired."

An Idea for Then and Now

What are the implications of the health center story for public policy, including issues specific to the centers, their relationship to public and private insurance, the opportunities posed by renewed activism at the community level, and the quest for tomorrow's heroes?

Should More Health Centers Be Funded?

A threshold policy question is whether the health center model should continue to be expanded with federal and state funds. The answer is "yes," based on the overwhelmingly positive record documented here and elsewhere. When they go head-to-head with the best health care systems, health centers hold their own or do better in terms of cost, quality, and value. Of particular interest are the studies showing that centers outperformed other Medicaid managed care providers on standard quality and outcome measures,[5] and that their users were significantly less likely than those of other providers to use hospitals and emergency rooms for conditions that might have been prevented by good ambulatory care.[6]

It is essential that health centers continue to compare well with other systems. But it's also important to look at how they are unique, because these special traits are under fire. Historically, centers were outsiders, a thorn in the side of establishment health care institutions and state/local power structures. They've come a long way in forging relationships through local networks and state political involvement. Yet traditional providers still covet the centers' grant subsidies and preferred reimbursement status, pushing for legislation that would not require consumer governance or anywhere near the concentration of uninsured and low-income people that health centers serve. When hospitals tried for similar legislation in 1978, Senator Ted Kennedy told them to "go the extra mile" and meet the governing board requirements, especially since some hospitals were working just fine with community boards.[7] Today, the very qualities that make health centers different mean that they are better able to meet the latest expectations.

Take the term "patient-centered services" that quality mavens like to use. Who does it better than health centers, with their painstaking devotion to respect and humanity? The way the centers treat patients is born of memories like those of L. C. Dorsey, whose plantation doctors rarely examined their patients, or Marsha Barros, who was shoved out of her wheelchair by a racist nurse at the old Boston City Hospital. When Mike Holloman asked a critical visitor why he thought the Ryan center's shiny new building was too nice for people who deserve the best, he said it all.

Then there's "consumer-driven care," too often a euphemism for schemes that end up costing the patient more. Economists like to talk about people "voting with their feet," but most people who use health centers don't have a great deal of choice. And even if they did have other options for where they get their care, is it better to let disgruntled patients walk out the door or invite them in to speak their piece? In conservative, blue-collar Boston, neighborhood residents on health center boards were so taken with the idea that they demanded autonomy from hospital sponsors years before it was mandated by the federal government. Centers give patients a real voice—a rarity in today's health care market.

Another expectation of some policy makers is that more "faith-based organizations" receive federal funds. Unfortunately, the term has somehow come to mean an exemption from federal standards and requirements. But what could be more faith based than the scores of health centers that started in church basements, or the missionaries and religious orders that sent doctors and nurses to centers in the nation's poorest areas, and even served as interim sponsors—without expecting that they, and not the duly empowered consumer board, would control the agenda?

What Do Health Centers Need to Thrive in the Future?

In order to thrive, the centers need funding streams to subsidize all services for the uninsured as well as social support or enabling services, typically not covered by insurance, for everyone. Such services tend to make care more efficient and effective. In 2004, although there were wide differences among centers, due in part to variations in coverage, federal grants averaged 24 percent of health center revenues and state, local, and private grants 13 percent.[8] As insurance continues to erode, grant subsidies need to increase simply to maintain the current level of service. This is an important investment: Although uninsured people generally are more likely to go without needed care and less likely to receive preventive services, these disadvantages are largely overcome for health center patients who lack insurance.[9] A major exception is specialty care. Nearly everywhere I visited, the centers were working overtime to assure access for their uninsured patients, but without specialty staff under their control, they inevitably fall short. This is confirmed by analysis of staffing patterns and published studies.[10] Federal authorities may want to consider some sort of matching program so that health centers can pay hospitals and private practices discounted fees for specialty care.

All this relates to existing centers and the patients they serve. In addition, as of 2004, implementation of President Bush's growth plan was roughly halfway complete. The patient population increased from 9.6 million in 2000 to an estimated 14 million in 2004.[11] The centers were on track to add perhaps another million patients. But starting with 2005, although the president's requested increases continued to be substantial, congressional appropriations slowed. To maintain quality and carry through with the second phase of the expansion, assuring a health center in every poor county, annual increases of at least $300 million, as provided in the early years of the initiative, will be required.

The centers also require assistance with capital needs and provider staffing. Although some health center associations have been creative in helping their members apply for financing and/or secure bond issues, construction is specifically excluded from federal operating grants. Policy makers might want to consider removing this prohibition.

Provider recruitment has taken a quantum leap over the early days, when centers were almost totally dependent on federally obligated or assigned providers from the National Health Service Corps (NHSC). Health centers and their associations have grown in sophistication, contracting with professional recruitment agencies and in some cases operating their own. In addition, practice in a health center has increased in popularity as schools and living conditions improved and relationships were forged (or reforged) with training institutions. The work environment compares favorably with managed care organizations, although compensation is still not as competitive. But the centers, especially those in more isolated rural areas, still need the NHSC and a parallel program obligating foreign-born physicians who trained in the U.S. to serve a term in an area with shortages of primary care providers under what is known as a J1 visa. For budgetary or other reasons, it is periodically proposed that these programs be eliminated, but their impact on health centers is considerable and should be considered a reason for at least maintenance of effort.

Administrative support is essential. Historically, health centers are indebted to champions within the government who took a personal interest in their success. To name just a few, they include the early antibureaucrats like Richard Boone, Sandy Kravitz, and Lee Schorr at OEO; the policy entrepreneurs at what was then the department of Health, Education and Welfare who started their own centers; Donald Rumsfeld, who went out of his way as OEO director to support the health center model in general and particular centers under political fire; Ed Martin, who prescribed the tough medicine that hurt some centers and saved many more; Karen Davis, who brought her economic expertise and network of academics and southern progressives to bear in support of the program; and managers like Marilyn Gaston, who broadened the centers' scope and awareness and highlighted elimination of health disparities, and Dick Bohrer, who somehow knew what was going on in every one of 900 organizations and loved to hold court as he offered advice and listened to their pleas for resources.

Some fear that much of the specialized hands-on knowledge of the past is gone now, victim of an administration that likes the program in the abstract but lacks the people and the will to nurture and develop its many parts. There are barely enough staffers to review reports and hand out checks, and project officers complain of limited travel funds. Bohrer joined the Public Health Service during the Vietnam War and stayed until 2003, rising to the rank of a two-star admiral and spending twenty years directing the health center program. He's especially concerned about the lack of support. "The agency is systematically eroding the program's infrastructure," he says. "People with experience are cut off as a resource, and carefully cultivated relationships throughout the department are left to lie fallow. The biggest problem is what will happen with Medicaid and Medicare, administered by a sister agency within the same department where contacts are essential."[12]

Cuts in staff and overhead look good to budget types, as does the enforced separation of decision making from people who might care too much. But expansion plans may be at risk, especially when the goal is to reach poverty-stricken counties that lack existing centers and other resources on which to build. Bohrer remembers the huge effort that went into the fourfold growth in the number of centers in the seventies, using consultants as well as central and regional office staff of the federal government. The ten regional offices—historically a force for both good and bad—no longer lead or develop or create; mainly, they conduct audits. The opportunity for a young Bill Hobson to ride the circuit, defying established tradition to establish new, comprehensive migrant health centers in the Northwest's agricultural valleys, is no longer there. And as one observer puts it, "Where would you find a Rose Forstner today?" The star of her own detective story on New York's Lower East Side, Forstner's stubborn curiosity uncovered fraud that no one else wanted to see, and she didn't stop there. She helped arrange a complicated shift in power from a criminally negligent organization to another center whose nontraditional leaders she trusted.

Health Centers and Insurance

Ted Kennedy is in a celebratory mood at the fortieth birthday party for Columbia Point, the nation's first operating health center. He kids the sponsors and the people in the audience and then turns serious: "I don't know what the nation would look like if we didn't have health centers, in terms of infant mortality, AIDS, TB, asthma. They came to your doorstep with every challenge and you said welcome." He continues: "My heart belongs to this movement. . . . As long as I have a voice I'll speak out for universal coverage and community health centers."

It's no accident that Kennedy and other knowledgeable policy makers link the two. We have seen that health centers and insurance coverage are complementary. Insurance alone does not overcome barriers to care related to a lack of providers, cultural differences, and outright discrimination. Even in countries where coverage is virtually universal, like Canada, policy makers are calling for support of delivery system expansion.[13]

Just as insurance needs a delivery system, health centers need insurance, especially now that they have a diversified revenue base and derive 57 percent of their budget from payments tied to individual patients.[14] Growth in Medicaid reimbursement under the Federally Qualified Health Center program, in particular, has enabled the centers to expand the numbers of insured and uninsured patients, and to build the critical mass needed to support such value-producing services as onsite labs, x-rays, and pharmacies.[15] But because they target low-income populations and serve all comers without regard to ability to pay, health centers are much more sensitive than other providers to cuts in public insurance, erosion of private coverage, and expansion of populations in need. Like canaries in a coal mine, they bear the brunt of massive demographic and economic changes—immigration, the increase of the service sector and its low-benefit jobs, and shrinking union strength.

Of course, these issues go far beyond their impact on health centers. It matters economically and morally whether the U.S. begins to treat health care as a right when every other developed nation has some form of universal coverage.

The huge geographic inequality in insurance, driven not only by the job market but also by demographics and widely varying state policies, is especially problematic. Federalism—reserving the bulk of policy decisions to the states—is a way of life in the U.S., but its importance may fade in the face of such great differences. Texas has the highest proportion of uninsured people—27.3 percent of the nonelderly—compared with the lowest proportion, 9.8 percent, in Minnesota. There is also a troubling racial/ethnic skew. In past years, the southeastern states, with their high numbers of low-income blacks and stingy Medicaid programs, were the worst trouble spots. Now at least some of these states have improved, and the lowest coverage rates are predominantly in states with large Hispanic populations. Of the eight states with over 20 percent of their nonelderly people uninsured, five are located along the southern border—Florida, Louisiana, Texas, New Mexico, and California. The other three are Oklahoma, with a large Native American population, and Nevada and Montana, both states where attitudes are still heavily influenced by the western culture of rugged individualism.[16] While this distribution may reflect negative attitudes about immigration, it raises a legitimate question: Should the burden of uninsured newcomers continue to rest on states and safety net providers, or should the federal government help equalize the situation? Failure to address this problem will have longer-term economic and business consequences.

The Broader Perspective

Health care for low-income, minority, and underserved people should also be seen in a wider context. The nation's gap between rich and poor has been growing since the 1970s,[17] it has become unfashionable to advance the concept of common responsibilities, and the market for health insurance—one of the last bastions of risk sharing—has become so segmented that we have high-cost "boutique" care for people who simply want to talk to their doctors when they are sick, and coverage for those with HIV/AIDS is sold as a "niche product."

Twice in the years between 2000 and 2005 it seemed that there was an opening toward the communitarian strain in American life, and just as quickly the door slammed shut. In the months following the terrorist attacks in 2001, people talked frequently about how they yearned for leaders with courage, for a sense of togetherness that seemed to have been lost, and for common sense in how to split and deal with problems that, taken together, are too much for anyone to bear.

Harvard professor Robert Putnam, who cataloged the erosion of togetherness and its impact on education, public safety, prosperity, and health in *Bowling Alone: The Collapse and Revival of American Community*,[18] urged that the post-9/11 focus on commonality be translated into "concrete policy initiatives that bridge the ethnic and class cleavages in our increasingly multicultural society."[19] But with unseemly speed, that surge of spirit was overshadowed by a controversial and expensive war in Iraq and contention over foreign policy. At home, we went about our separate lives.

Then came Hurricane Katrina in 2005, the searing photos and videos of desolation, with hundreds of thousands of people left behind, figuratively and in a nightmare of reality. That was followed by a spate of questions as to whether the nation was ready, after forty years, to rediscover poverty. Again, the spotlight shifted quickly away from the problems of the poor. Almost as a cruel hoax, the already stretched resources of social programs were cut even further to pay for disaster relief and help reduce deficits. Early in 2006 Congress voted $93 billion in savings over the next ten years, with 27 percent of that coming from Medicaid cuts—despite a recent warning from the nonpartisan Congressional Budget Office (CBO) that this will cause 65,000 enrollees, including 39,000 children, to lose their coverage; thirteen million low-income people will face increased cost sharing, including ten million who will actually have services reduced. And the CBO found that expected savings were likely to be reduced by counterproductive increases in emergency room and chronic disease care. The wealthy, already enriched by multiple tax cuts, bore little or no share of the burden.[20]

It didn't look as if a new golden age were coming anytime soon. Jack Geiger has been struck by the aptness of a book called *The Unsteady March: The Rise and Decline of Racial Equality in America.*[21] Only in the wake of large-scale war, the authors say, has the U.S. been able to move toward equality—the contribution of the minority group becomes clear, inclusion is enhanced, and protest movements succeed in pressing reforms.

Back to the Community

While broader shifts in resources are ultimately called for, in the short term, efforts at the community level may offer the greatest opportunity for action. Communities are where healing takes place, people recognize the importance of interrelationships, and the scale is small enough that modest resources have significant payoff. Health centers can be one point of departure. Geiger says that if he had his way, not only would there be universal health insurance and more health centers, but the centers would be funded for more nonhealth activities appropriate to the needs of their particular neighborhoods.[22] Richard Boone, who helped develop the concept of citizen participation and launch the early OEO programs, sees a role for the centers in renewed and expanded training of paraprofessionals and involvement of residents in improving the community.[23]

On a warm summer evening upward of eighty young researchers are gathered at a conference center near Leesburg, Virginia. Doctoral candidates and postdoctoral fellows, their diverse backgrounds include epidemiology, clinical medicine, environmental science, sociology, and economics. They are focused on the disturbing disparities in health status that continue to plague the U.S. Medical expenditures consistently exceed those of all other developed countries,[24] and in 2004 approached $6,300 per person.[25] But the risk of mortality in this nation is still three times as great for the poor compared with those who are relatively well off,[26] and infant deaths are still twice as prevalent for black babies as for white babies.[27] In turn, these ongoing disparities in the face of improvement in other countries help drive our declining international position. In 1960 the U.S. had the eleventh lowest infant mortality rate among developed nations; in 2002 its position had dropped to twenty-eighth.[28]

The researchers' meeting begins with a film that features an earnest young man who cautions: "Health care alone is not the point. That would be like putting on a band-aid and sending our patients back home to the same conditions that made them sick in the first place." A quote from state-of-the-art research on the social determinants of health? Not exactly. The film—grainy and homemade—is more than thirty-five years old. Set in the Delta Health Center in Mississippi, it contains graphic scenes of unrelenting poverty—stoop labor, ten or twelve people crowding into a tiny shack. A nurse is seen bathing a newborn in a field; some people are digging wells, attending classes, learning to run a food cooperative. The voice is that of then director Geiger. After the film, he's joined by John Hatch and L. C. Dorsey, and the three discuss the center's approach and its relevance for today's policies.

At the end of the session, the audience stands and applauds for a full five minutes. They are struck by how much the Mississippi experience parallels the latest studies on what makes us healthy. The takeaway message is clear: Academics may argue over what influences health the most—medical care, personal behavior, racial disparities, or social, economic, and environmental factors. People who live and work in communities know that these factors are inextricably linked. You can't have a healthy society unless you pay attention to all of them.

Tomorrow's Heroes

Notwithstanding the fact that some health center directors haven't trained their replacements, the question of tomorrow's heroes is a central one, on the minds of many. At every level, the older leaders I interviewed speak of their experience in glowing terms. "The community health center movement—it's been an absolute love affair my whole life," says national association president Tom Van Coverden. "The energy, the leadership, the people steeped in traditions of civil rights and helping others, social justice and positive action."[29] Hatch, who moved on from Mississippi to organize prevention efforts through North Carolina's churches, says the health center experience "was the richest part of my professional life. People who had dreams for their children saw them come true."[30]

Yet they also fear that young people lack the same level of commitment. Progress has brought the burgeoning health field superbly trained scientists, researchers, managers, and practitioners—a growing though still insufficient proportion of them minorities. Many of these young men and women are unaware of how health centers and the people who founded them anchored their work in historic social movements. Others may be carried away by the understandable lure of professional status and hefty salaries. Indeed, the skills and management sophistication needed to run a modern-day health center can be all consuming. But the centers didn't survive and grow into the nation's largest primary care network without challenging public health orthodoxy, medical sovereignty, and entrenched bureaucracy. And they won't thrive in future years unless they continue to do so.

"Health centers need to be recast as a mission—the moral bulwark in a collapsing system of care that is abandoning the poor," Geiger believes. He is buoyed by periodic mail and speaking invitations from medical students and young physicians who are fascinated by the program's early history and its relevance for today. One fourth-year student had recently followed Geiger's suggestion to spend time at the Delta Health Center in Mississippi and then returned to spread the word by organizing a course for other students on physician advocacy.[31]

Hatch says that despite an atmosphere that is less supportive of social change, "some people do have that spark. There are urgent public issues that capture my attention—situations that are destructive of society, perhaps unwittingly." One is a justice system that is decimating the young black male population and returning them to communities as criminals and deviants. Another is the large hog and chicken farms wreaking havoc in once beautiful but resource-poor rural areas and posing huge public health concerns. He goes on: "I never met a community that didn't want to improve how it lives. But they may need help in connecting the dots for policy makers, and that's where young academics come in."[32]

Thus efforts to support scholar-activists and link them to health centers and communities may be one place to start. The W. K. Kellogg Foundation sponsors Geiger fellowships on Capitol Hill and supports pre- and postdoctoral scholars working on health disparities. "The model for action was there in the health centers of the sixties," a participant in one of these programs says. "I am determined to honor this legacy through my own work." Health centers once worked closely with researchers. In particular, the faculty members hired by the Tufts medical school to study and support the first centers helped give birth to the field of applied anthropology and presaged the concepts of community-based participatory research, giving ownership of results to the study subjects. A core of young academics focused on modern-day health centers could address such topics as the social determinants of health, the impact of neighborhoods and the physical environment, the role of governance and community empowerment, and the use of research to advance the lot of patients and their families.

A major task will be passing on the health center legacy to new managers and executives. It's on the agenda of a program named for Geiger and Count Gibson at George Washington University. "Leadership and succession are the driving force in my thinking and may be our biggest test," according to Sara Rosenbaum, the health policy department chair who spearheaded development of the program.[33] As of early 2006 current health center leaders were doing stints as visiting scholars, and the content for students was under development. "There's a lot of conversation but no answers yet," Bohrer says. He sees opportunities in mentoring and knowledge transfer.

During the early civil rights movement, before the culture wars, young people learned about hope and redemption from mythic leaders. They used to say they ended up gaining much more than they gave. Is there a modern-day counterpart? Don Sykes, whose community action experience parallels that of the early health center leaders, wants to start an institute where young people "who have the skills but lack the fire" can learn from the older generation.[34]

Courage and resilience were hallmarks of the first heroes of community health—men and women who persevered forty years ago in the face of far greater personal odds than those most of us can imagine. I know that even if we could bottle the best of those heady and exciting times, it wouldn't quite fit in the twenty-first century. But there are some timeless principles that are more important now than ever before: The courage to move against the grain. The knowledge that communities of all kinds matter. And a lasting commitment to make the world a better place.

Notes

Chapter 1. Heroes of Community Health

1. For early health center history, see Alice Sardell, *The U.S. Experiment in Social Medicine: The Community Health Center Program, 1965–1986* (Pittsburgh: University of Pittsburgh Press, 1988).

2. Health centers reported serving 13.1 million people in 2004, according to Bureau of Primary Health Care, Health Resources and Services Administration, U.S. Department of Health and Human Services, Uniform Data System, http://bphc.hrsa .gov/uds/2004data/nattrend.htm, accessed November 30, 2005. In addition, there were roughly 700,000 users of newly funded capacity (not reported in their first year), according to Daniel Hawkins, National Association of Community Health Centers, communication with author, January 19, 2005.

3. See, for example, "Transcript of President Bush's Message to Congress on His Budget Proposal," *New York Times*, February 28, 2001.

4. For a detailed, ground-up history of the civil rights movement in the fifties and sixties, see Taylor Branch's three-volume series, *Parting the Waters: America in the King Years 1954–63* (New York: Simon and Schuster, 1988); *Pillar of Fire: America in the King Years 1963–65* (New York: Simon and Schuster, 1998); and *At Canaan's Edge: America in the King Years 1965–68* (New York: Simon and Schuster, 2006).

5. An excellent, though uncritical, description of the "politics of lifestyle" can be found in David Brooks, *Bobos in Paradise: The New Upper Class and How They Got There* (New York: Simon and Schuster, 2000).

6. Peter Edelman, *Searching for America's Heart: RFK and the Renewal of Hope* (New York: Houghton Mifflin, 2001), 80–81.

7. Robert F. Clark, *The War on Poverty: History, Selected Programs and Ongoing Impact* (Lanham, Md.: University Press of America, 2002), 9–60.

8. See, for example, Robert E. Rector, *How "Poor" Are America's Poor?* Backgrounder No. 791 (Washington, D.C.: Heritage Foundation, 1990). There were also critiques, particularly in the more expansive early days, from those who believed that the War on Poverty did not go far enough in empowering the poor and righting class differences. See, for example, Christopher Jencks, "Johnson vs. Poverty," *New Republic*, March 28, 1964.

9. Clark, *War on Poverty*. See also Michael Harrington, *The Other America: Poverty in the United States* (New York: Macmillan, 1962).

10. Richard Boone, interview by author, Santa Barbara, Calif., November 9, 2004, and subsequent communications.

11. Sanford Kravitz, telephone interview by author, September 6, 2002, and subsequent communications. For a discussion of concepts behind opportunity theory, see Richard A. Cloward and Lloyd E. Ohlin, *Delinquency and Opportunity: A Theory of Delinquent Gangs* (Glencoe, Ill.: Free Press, 1960).

12. Boone, interview and subsequent communications.

13. Clark, *War on Poverty*, 28–30.

14. Michael L. Gillette, *Launching the War on Poverty: An Oral History* (New York: Twayne, 1996), 84–85.

15. H. Jack Geiger, telephone interview by author, September 20, 2002, and subsequent communications.

16. Richard A. Couto, *Ain't Gonna Let Nobody Turn Me Round: The Pursuit of Racial Justice in the Rural South* (Philadelphia: Temple University Press, 1991), ch. 8; augmented by author's conversations about management style with former OEO staffers.

17. Boone, interview and subsequent communications.

18. H. Jack Geiger, "Community Health Centers: Health Care as an Instrument of Social Change," in Victor Sidel and Ruth Sidel, eds., *Reforming Medicine: Lessons of the Last Quarter Century* (New York: Pantheon, 1984), cited in Sardell, *U.S. Experiment in Social Medicine*, 66–67.

19. Lisbeth B. Schorr, with Daniel Schorr, *Within Our Reach: Breaking the Cycle of Disadvantage* (New York: Doubleday, 1988), 131.

20. For a thorough account of the struggle to integrate hospitals, see David Barton Smith, *Health Care Divided: Race and Healing a Nation* (Ann Arbor: University of Michigan Press, 1999).

21. Sidney Kark and Emily Kark, *Promoting Community Health: From Pholela to Jerusalem* (Johannesburg: Witwatersrand University Press, 1999).

22. Schorr, *Within Our Reach*, 130–131.

23. Ibid.

24. H. Jack Geiger, "The First Community Health Centers: A Model of Enduring Value," *Journal of Ambulatory Care Management* 28, no. 4 (2205): 213–320.

25. Kravitz, interview and subsequent communications.

26. Geiger, interview.

27. Schorr, *Within Our Reach*, 32.

28. Couto, *Ain't Gonna Let Nobody Turn Me Round*, ch. 8; Schorr, *Within Our Reach*, 132; Sardell, *U.S. Experiment in Social Medicine*, 66–67.

29. Jude Thomas May and Peter Kong-ming New, Transcripts for Oral History Project (Washington, D.C.: NACHC, 1974–1977), cited in Sardell, *U.S. Experiment in Social Medicine*, 52; Sardell, *U.S. Experiment in Social Medicine*, 68–73.

30. David Blumenthal, "Out OEO-ing OEO: Institutional Innovation in the Public Health Service" (Master's thesis, Department of Government, Harvard University, 1970), cited in Sardell, *U.S. Experiment in Social Medicine*, 68–73.

31. The projection of 1,000 centers is from a 1967 HEW planning document cited by Karen Davis and Cathy Schoen, *Health and the War on Poverty: A Ten-Year Appraisal* (Washington, D.C.: Brookings Institution, 1978), 163. Blumenthal, in "Out OEO-ing OEO," mentions a smaller projection of 600 centers.

32. William D. Hobson, interview by author, Los Angeles, November 5, 2004.

33. Richard N. Goodwin, *Remembering America: A Voice from the Sixties* (New York: Little, Brown, 1988), 417–427, 456.

34. Schorr, *Within Our Reach*, 131.

35. Sardell, *U.S. Experiment in Social Medicine*, 64–66; Geiger, "Community Health Centers."

36. Couto, *Ain't Gonna Let Nobody Turn Me Round*, ch. 8

37. Subsequent problems with hospitals: from the author's experience with administration of health centers; this was also a common theme in interviews with health center leaders.

38. Office of Economic Opportunity, Health Services, *The Comprehensive Neighborhood Health Services Program: Guidelines*, OEO Guidance No. 6128–1 (Washington, D.C.: Executive Office of the President, March 1970).

39. Couto, *Ain't Gonna Let Nobody Turn Me Round*, 264–266.

40. Sardell, *U.S. Experiment in Social Medicine*, 77–78.

41. Couto, *Ain't Gonna Let Nobody Turn Me Round*, 282–283.

42. Clark, *War on Poverty*, 206.

43. Couto, *Ain't Gonna Let Nobody Turn Me Round*, 282–283.

44. Paul Starr, *The Social Transformation of American Medicine* (New York: Basic Books, 1982), 396.

45. Couto, *Ain't Gonna Let Nobody Turn Me Round*, 282–283; Sardell, *U.S. Experiment in Social Medicine*, 81.

46. Clark, *War on Poverty*, 64–68.

47. Sardell, *U.S. Experiment in Social Medicine*, 86–89. Until the legislation was enacted in 1975, the program was known as Neighborhood Health Centers; the new law changed the name to Community Health Centers. In most places throughout the book I refer to the "health center program" to avoid confusion. Kennedy's comment on governance provisions is from *Roll Call*, interview with Senator Edward M. Kennedy, February 28, 2002.

48. Ann Zuvekas, "Cutback Decisionmaking: The Community Health Center Program" (Ph.D. diss., George Washington University, 1984), 47–50.

49. Except where otherwise noted, this section is from the author's personal experience. From 1977 to 1980, I served at HEW, later HHS, as director of health services and resources analysis office of the deputy assistant secretary for planning and evaluation. For an understanding of knowledge and interest in health centers from this office, see Davis and Schoen, *Health and the War on Poverty*, 161–202; and U.S. Department of Health, Education and Welfare, Office of the Deputy Assistant Secretary for Planning and Evaluation, Health, *National Health Insurance Papers* (Washington, D.C.: U.S. Department of Health and Human Services, 1980).

50. Rural Health Clinic Services Act of 1977 (P.L. 95–210).

51. Sardell, *U.S. Experiment in Social Medicine*, 149–161.

52. Ibid., 174, 189.

53. Clark, *War on Poverty*, 70–71.

54. Bonnie Lefkowitz, "Short Term Options for Categorical Health Grant Programs," in *Working Papers on Major Budget and Program Issues in Selected Health Programs* (Washington, D.C.: U.S. Congressional Budget Office, 1976).

55. Daniel Hawkins, interviews by author, Washington, D.C., September 9 and November 5, 2002.

56. David A. V. Reynolds, "An Analysis of the Political and Economic Viability of Community Health Centers: Implications for Their Future" (Ph.D. diss., University of Michigan, 1999), 6–31.

57. Jacqueline Leifer, telephone interview by author, February 16, 2006.

58. Reynolds, "Community Health Centers," 6–31.

59. Tom Van Coverden, interview by author, Bethesda, Md., August 16, 2002; Hawkins, interviews.

60. Zuvekas, "Cutback Decisionmaking," 51–62, 93–156.

61. Bonnie Lefkowitz and Jennifer Todd, "An Overview: Community Health Centers at the Crossroads," *Journal of Ambulatory Care Management* 2, no. 4 (1991): 1–12.

62. Hawkins, interviews.

63. Institute of Medicine, *America's Health Care Safety Net: Intact but Endangered* (Washington, D.C.: National Academies Press, 2000), 120–121.

64. Except where otherwise noted, this section is drawn from the author's personal experience. I served as cochair of the "cluster" on underserved populations and preventive health for the Clinton health care reform task force, and from 1993 to 1999

at HHS as associate bureau director for data, evaluation, analysis, and research for the Bureau of Primary Health Care, Health Resources and Services Administration, where the community health center program is administered.

65. White House Health Care Reform Task Force, *Underserved Populations and Preventive Health: Delivery System Efforts Under Health Care Reform*, Tollgate 5, Staff Working Paper, March 1993.

66. U.S. House of Representatives, Health Security Act, H.R. 3600, September 20, 1993, Title III, Subtitle E—Health Services for Medically Underserved Populations (health center and related support), and Title I, Subtitle F—Federal Responsibilities (creation and review of essential community providers).

67. Theda Skocpol, *Boomerang: Clinton's Health Security Effort and the Turn against Government in U.S. Politics* (New York: Norton, 1996).

68. Daniel Hawkins, communication to author, October 28, 2002.

69. Hawkins, interviews.

70. "Transcript of President Bush's Message to Congress on His Budget Proposal," *New York Times*, February 28, 2001.

71. "Transcript of President Bush's State of the Union Message," *New York Times*, February 2, 2005.

72. National Association of Community Health Centers, *Washington Update* Hotline, Week of December 13, 2004.

73. National Association of Community Health Centers, "2005 Year in Review," Press Release, January 3, 2006.

74. National Association of Community Health Centers, *Washington Update* Hotline, Week of February 13, 2006.

75. U.S. Office of Management and Budget, Program Assessment, www.expectmore.gov, accessed February 13, 2006.

76. Larry T. Patton, "Community Health Centers at 25: A Retrospective Look at the First 10 Years," *Journal of Ambulatory Care Management* 3, no. 4 (1990): 13–21.

77. Clark, *War on Poverty*, 298.

78. Hawkins, communication.

79. Nicholas Lemann, "The Myth of Community Development," *New York Times Magazine*, January 9, 1994.

80. Massachusetts League of Community Health Centers, *Community Health Centers as Economic Engines: An Overview of Their Impact on Massachusetts Communities and Families* (Boston: Massachusetts League of Community Health Centers, October 2003).

81. Henry Bonilla, "The Heart of Health Care," column for local Texas papers, July 20, 2005; Office of Senator Kit Bond, "Bond Pledges to Continue Fight for Community Health Centers," Press Release, August 25, 2005.

82. Bureau of Primary Health Care, Uniform Data System, http://bphc.hrsa.gov/uds/2004data/nattrend.htm, accessed November 30, 2005.

83. Ann Zuvekas, "Health Centers and the Health Care System," *Journal of Ambulatory Care Management* 28, no. 4 (2005): 331–339.

84. Kaiser Commission on Medicaid and the Uninsured, November 2005 Update.

85. National Association of Community Health Centers, *A Nation's Health at Risk: A National and State Report on America's 36 Million People without a Regular Health Care Provider* (Washington, D.C.: National Association of Community Health Centers, 2004).

86. Institute of Medicine, *Unequal Treatment: Confronting Racial and Ethnic Disparities in Health Care* (Washington, D.C.: National Academies Press, 2002).

87. See note 2. In addition, Hawkins estimates that one million people use FQHC "look-alikes," or centers that meet requirements but do not receive federal grants.

88. Bureau of Primary Health Care, Uniform Data System, http://bphc.hrsa.gov/uds/2004data/nattrend.htm, accessed November 30, 2005.

89. Major effectiveness studies include: Barbara Starfield et al., "Costs vs. Quality in Different Types of Primary Care Settings," *Journal of the American Medical Association* 272, no. 24 (1994): 1903–1908; Lee Partridge, *The APHSA Medicaid HEDIS Database Project, Report for the Third Project Year*, (Washington, D.C.: American Public Human Services Association, December 2001); M. E. Stuart and Donald M. Steinwachs, "Patient-Mix Differences among Ambulatory Care Providers and Their Effects on Utilization and Payments for Maryland Medicaid Users," *Medical Care* 31, no. 12 (1992): 119–137; Ann Zuvekas, Kathy McNamara, and Caryn Bernstein, "Measuring the Primary Care Experiences of Low-Income and Minority Patients," *Journal of Ambulatory Care Management* 22, no. 4 (1999): 63–78; Jerrilyn Regan, Bonnie Lefkowitz, and Marilyn Gaston, "Cancer Screening among Community Health Center Women: Eliminating the Gaps," *Journal of Ambulatory Care Management* 22, no. 4 (1999): 45–52; Marilyn Falik et al., "Ambulatory Care Sensitive Hospitalizations and Emergency Visits: Experiences of Medicaid Patients Using Federally Qualified Health Centers," *Medical Care* 39, no. 6 (2000): 551–561; Marilyn Falik et al., "Comparative Effectiveness of FQHCs as Regular Source of Care: Application of Sentinel ACSC Events as Performance Measures," *Journal of Ambulatory Care Management*, forthcoming, 2006; Marshall H. Chin et al., "Improving Diabetes Care in Midwest Community Health Centers with the Health Disparities Collaborative," *Diabetes Care* 27, no. 1 (2004): 2–8. For an overview of effectiveness studies, see Michelle Proser, "Deserving the Spotlight: Health Centers Provide High-Quality and Cost-Effective Care," *Journal of Ambulatory Care Management* 28, no. 4 (2005): 321–330.

Chapter 2. Mississippi

1. Mississippi's age-adjusted death rate, 1,035 per 100,000 people, was higher than that of any other state for the period 2000–2002. The national rate was 853 per 100,000 people. National Center for Health Statistics, *Health United States, 2005* (Hyattsville, Md.: National Center for Health Statistics, 2005), table 28.

2. L. C. Dorsey, interview by author, Itta Bena, Miss., June 26, 2002, and subsequent communications. The story about her father's reckoning is from her presentation at the W. K. Kellogg Symposium on Health of the Nation: Moving from Disparities to Health and Welfare Policy, June 19, 2002; her father's accompanying her to the school bus is from H. Jack Geiger, "On Accepting the Gustave Lienhard Award," address to Institute of Medicine, October 12, 1998.

3. N. Maxwell, "The Ailing Poor: Medical Team Combats Negroes' Dismal Health in Mississippi Delta," *Wall Street Journal*, January 14, 1969.

4. Ollye Shirley, interview by author, Washington, D.C., March 27, 2002.

5. Aaron Shirley, interviews by author, Washington, D.C., April 29, 2002, and Jackson, Miss., June 27, 2002, and subsequent communications.

6. Robert Smith, interview by author, Jackson, Miss., June 27, 2002, and subsequent communication.

7. The 1960 infant mortality rates in Mississippi and its counties provided by Mississippi Department of Health, communication to author; national rate from National Center for Health Statistics, *Health United States, 2001* (Hyattsville, Md.: National Center for Health Statistics, 2001), table 23.

8. U.S. Census information on housing in Mississippi cited in Geiger, "First Community Health Centers," 313–320.

9. Geiger, interview and subsequent communications.

10. Maxwell, "Ailing Poor."

11. Helen Barnes, interview by author, Jackson, Miss., June 27, 2002, and subsequent communication.

12. Hatch's explanation of hunger, unemployment, and results of job training are from his presentation at the W. K. Kellogg Symposium on Health of the Nation: Moving from Disparities to Health and Welfare Policy, June 19, 2002. The results of the center's job training and career ladder programs are from Geiger, "On Accepting Lienhard Award."

13. James (Andy) Anderson, interview by author, Jackson, Miss., June 28, 2002.

14. G. B. Baldwin, "Center Built Despite Obstacles," *Jackson Clarion Ledger*, August 26, 2000.

15. Ibid.

16. Kenneth W. Clawson, "U.S. Sues Mississippi to Free Health Funds," *Washington Post*, March 3, 1971.

17. Geiger, "On Accepting Lienhard Award."

18. Bonnie Lefkowitz, "From New York to Jackson . . . Stoned on Soul," *Manhattan Tribune*, May 15, 1971.

19. Jackson-Hinds's leadership, teen programs, and visit by federal officials are from author's recollection of site visit in 1979. I was one of the HHS representatives on the visiting committee.

20. Information about federal demands for reorganization of Delta Health Center: author's recollection.

21. Ann Zuvekas, "Community Training and Services in a Medical Mall: Missed Opportunities," paper prepared for Third National Primary Care Conference, February 26–28, 1997.

22. Author's visits to Jackson Medical Mall and new facility of Jackson-Hinds health center, June 28, 2002.

23. W. H. Frey, "Census 2000 Shows Large Black Return to the South, Reinforcing the Region's 'White-Black' Demographic Profile," Institute for Social Research, University of Michigan, 2001.

24. National Association of Community Health Centers, www.nachc.com, accessed December 2005.

25. Sister Trinita Eddington, interview by author, Jackson, Miss., June 27, 2002.

26. Kaiser Commission on Medicaid and the Uninsured, November 2005 Update.

Chapter 3. Boston

1. James W. Hunt, interview by author, Boston, August 15, 2002, and subsequent communications.

2. Tristram Blake, interview by author, Boston, August 13, 2002.

3. Infant mortality and tuberculosis in Boston's South End from Governing Board of the South End Health Center and Pediatric Service of Boston City Hospital, "Outline of Proposal for a Childrens' Clinic for the South End of Boston," 1968. Comparable national infant mortality from Davis and Schoen, *Health and the War on Poverty*, 37, table 2–4.

4. Dale Young, *A Promise Kept: Boston's Neighborhood Health Centers* (Boston: Trustees of Health and Hospitals, 1982), 42.

5. Lack of prenatal care in Boston's North End from Jack Cradock, interview by author, East Boston, Mass., August 14, 2002; comparable national figure for 1970 from

National Center for Health Statistics, *Health United States, 1998* (Hyattsville, Md.: National Center for Health Statistics, 1998), table 6.

6. Problems in Boston neighborhood from 1965 grant application for Tufts Comprehensive Community Health Action Program, H. Jack Geiger, communication to author, January 2006.

7. Jean Hunt, interview by author, Boston, August 15, 2002.

8. James Taylor, interview by author, East Boston, Mass., August 13, 2002.

9. Herbert Gleason, interview by author, Boston, August 14, 2002.

10. Marsha Barros, interview by author, Boston, August 16, 2002.

11. James W. Hunt, "Community Health Centers' Impact on the Political and Economic Environment: The Massachusetts Example," *Journal of Ambulatory Care Management* 28, no. 4 (2005): 340–347.

12. H. Jack Geiger, interviews by author, telephone August 15, 2004; Boston, November 21, 2005; and subsequent communications.

13. Jeffrey Salloway, interview by author, Alton Bay, N.H., August 5, 2002, and subsequent communication.

14. For example, Sardell, *U.S. Experiment in Social Medicine*, and Couto, *Ain't Gonna Let Nobody Turn Me Round*, acknowledge extensive use of the May-New interviews as background and directly.

15. Daniel Driscoll, "Neighborhood Health Centers: Case Studies in Professional Domination" (Master's thesis, Cornell University, 1972).

16. Adam Clymer, *Edward M. Kennedy: A Biography* (New York: HarperCollins, 1999), 86–87.

17. Young, *Promise Kept*, Appendix B, 20, 27.

18. Ibid., 41–45.

19. James Hooley, interview by author, Boston, August 12, 2002, and subsequent communication.

20. Gerald Hass, interview by author, Boston, August 13, 2002.

21. Mel Scovell, interview by author, Boston, August 13, 2002.

22. Young, *Promise Kept*, Appendix B, 33.

23. Ibid., Appendix B, 10.

24. Cradock, interview.

25. Daniel Driscoll, interview by author, Dorchester, Mass., August 14, 2002.

26. Hunt, "Community Health Centers' Impact."

27. Kaiser Commission on Medicaid and the Uninsured, November 2005 Update.

28. Anita Crawford, telephone interview by author, October 3, 2005.

29. Van Coverden, interview.

30. James W. Hunt, interview; Hunt, "Community Health Centers' Impact."

Chapter 4. The South Carolina Low Country

1. Chicora Foundation, "Indian and Freemen Occupation at the Fish Haul Site (38BU805)," Beaufort County, South Carolina, Research Series 7, Columbia, S.C.

2. Emory Campbell, interview by author, St. Helena Island, S.C., February 13, 2002.

3. County data for 1960 from Geospatial and Statistical Data Center, University of Virginia Library, geostat@virginia.edu, accessed February 1, 2006; comparable national data for 1960 from U.S. Census, accessed through same Web site.

4. Tom Barnwell, interviews by author, Ridgeland, S.C., February 13, 2002; conference call, December 2005; telephone, February 10, 2006; and subsequent communication.

5. Roland Gardner, interviews by author, Washington, D.C., March 2001; Ridgeland, S.C., February 13, 2002; conference call, December 2005; and subsequent communications.

6. Louis Dore, interview by author, conference call, December 2005.

7. Ginnie Kozak, "Beaufort's History: Multifaceted and Fascinating," in *Destination Beaufort* (Beaufort, S.C.: Beaufort Regional Chamber of Commerce, 2006).

8. Omar Ford, "Center Continues Historic Evolution," *Beaufort Gazette*, June 15, 2003.

9. *Hunger U.S.A.: A Report by the Citizens' Board of Inquiry into Hunger and Malnutrition in the United States* (Boston: Beacon Press, 1968).

10. Ibid., 18, 23.

11. David Nolan, "The Hunger Doctor," *New York Review of Books*, March 11, 1971.

12. Ibid.; Harry Golden, *Nation*, November 25, 1968.

13. Gardner, interviews.

14. Carolyn Click, *Peace Corps Online*, November 22, 2004.

15. U.S. Senate, Hearings before the Select Committee on Nutrition and Human Needs, Ninety-first Congress, First Session, Part Four, South Carolina, Washington, D.C., February 18–20, 1969, testimony of Thomas Barnwell and William Grant, 1184–1189.

16. Campbell, interview.

17. Gardner, interviews.

18. Thaddeous Coleman, interview by author, Ridgeland, S.C., February 13, 2002; conference call, December 2005; and subsequent communication.

19. Beaufort-Jasper-Hampton Comprehensive Health Services Health Care Plan Update submitted to HHS Health Resources and Services Administration, 2005.

20. U.S. Census QuickFacts, http://quickfacts.census.gov, accessed November 23, 2005.

21. Aida Rogers, "The Island Everyone Knows," *Sandlapper, The Magazine of South Carolina*, www.sandlapper.org, accessed September 15, 2005.

22. U.S. Census QuickFacts.

23. Leslie Berger, "Retired Doctors, Retired Nurses, Very Busy Clinics," *New York Times*, November 14, 2005.

24. National Center for Health Statistics, *Health United States, 1998*, table 24; *Health United States, 2004* (Hyattsville, Md.: National Center for Health Statistics, 2004), table 23.

25. Kaiser Commission on Medicaid and the Uninsured, November 2005 Update.

26. Lathran Woodard, telephone interview by author, February 2006.

27. Sandra Walsh, "10,000 Babies Later, Noted Doctor Retires," *Beaufort Gazette*, October 20, 2005.

28. Rogers, "Island Everyone Knows."

29. Tim Donnelly, "Activist Being Roasted Friday," *Beaufort Gazette*, January 31, 2005; Omar Ford, "Health Officials Await Prostate Cancer Study Results," *Beaufort Gazette*, December 29, 2003.

30. Omar Ford, "More Minorities Take Jobs in Management," *Beaufort Gazette*, December 16, 2002.

Chapter 5. New York

1. Ann Zuvekas, communication to author.

2. New York City Department of Health and Mental Hygiene, Bureau of Vital Statistics, reports by health center district for 1960.

3. Paul Torrens, interview by author, Los Angeles, November 4, 2004.

4. Catherine Krouser, interview by author, New York, November 13, 2002.

5. Arnaldo Barron, interview by author, New York, November 12, 2002.

6. Julio (Jay) Bellber, interview by author, New York, November 11, 2002, and subsequent communication.

7. History prepared for William F. Ryan Community Health Center management retreat, April 4–6, 2003.

8. New York regional staff preference for professionals and institutions: author's recollection as a federal official.

9. Robin Finn, "Public Lives: At Health Center, Fighting Obesity Is No Joke," *New York Times*, March 12, 2004.

10. Barbra Minch, interview by author, New York, November 12, 2002, and subsequent communications.

11. Holloman's background is from Bellber, interview; and Minch, interview.

12. Comments of federal officials: author's recollection.

13. New York City Department of Health and Mental Hygiene, Bureau of Vital Statistics, reports by health center district for 1985.

14. Victor Papa, interview by author, New York, November 14, 2002.

15. Federal-state meeting about NENA: author's recollection; I represented HHS.

16. Kathy Gruber, interview by author, New York, November 14, 2002.

17. History prepared for Ryan management retreat.

18. Bobbie Maniece-Harrison, interview by author, New York, November 13, 2002.

19. Will Murphy, interview by author, New York, November 14, 2002.

20. Maria Lugo, interview by author, New York, November 14, 2002.

21. Kaiser Commission on Medicaid and the Uninsured, November 2005 Update.

22. Judy Wessler, interview by author, New York, July 16, 2004, and subsequent communication.

23. Data on bad debt and charity care burden for individual hospitals from New York State Department of Health, obtained through United Hospital Fund of New York.

24. William F. Ryan Community Health Center data prepared for federal Uniform Data System report, 2005.

25. Kenneth Raske, interview by author, New York, September 13, 2004.

26. Tom Robbins, "Hospital Holiday," *Village Voice*, May 28–June 3, 2003.

27. Commission on the Public's Health System, "CHCCDP: Are We Getting Our Money's Worth: Monitoring the Use of Community Health Care Conversion Demonstration Project Funds," April 2003.

28. James C. Robinson, "The Curious Conversion of Empire Blue Cross: In New York It's All Politics, All the Time," *Health Affairs* 22, no. 4 (July/August 2003): 100–118.

29. Ibid.; Michael Cooper, "In Conversion of Insurer, Contracts Go to Insiders," *New York Times*, October 1, 2005.

30. Richard N. Gottfried, interview by author, New York, July 16, 2004.

31. George Lowe, interview by author, New York, July 16, 2004.

32. Association for Community Affiliated Plans, representing health center plans and plans with similar ownership.

33. "Fidelis Care, CenterCare Sign Agreement," Press Release, Fidelis Care, June 13, 2005.

34. New York City Department of Health and Mental Hygiene, Bureau of Vital Statistics, reports by heath center district for 2004.

35. Albert Amateau, "A Battle Over an Orchard, But Chekhov's Not Involved," *Villager*, February 23–March 1, 2005.

Chapter 6. The Rio Grande Valley of Texas

1. Paula Gomez, interviews by author, telephone, February 20, 2003; Brownsville, Tex., March 11–14, 2003; and subsequent communications.
2. S. Dillon, "Profits Raise Pressure on U.S. Owned Factories in Mexican Border Zone," *New York Times*, February 15, 2001.
3. U.S. Bureau of Labor Statistics, www.bls.gov/oes, accessed October 31, 2005.
4. Alix Flores, interview by author, Brownsville, Tex., March 13, 2003.
5. Kaiser Commission on Medicaid and the Uninsured, November 2005 Update.
6. Gomez, interviews.
7. David Montejano, *Anglos and Mexicans in the Making of Texas, 1836–1986* (Austin: University of Texas Press, 1987), 8–9, 116–128.
8. Domingo Gonzalez, interview by author, Brownsville, Tex., March 11, 2003.
9. Montejano, *Anglos and Mexicans*, 159–196.
10. U.S. Census, 2000.
11. Gonzalez, interview.
12. Texas State Department of Health, Vital Statistics for 1960.
13. Luisa Franzini, John C. Ribble, and Arlene M. Keddie, "Understanding the Hispanic Paradox," in Thomas A. LaViest, ed., *Race, Ethnicity and Health: A Public Health Reader* (San Francisco: Jossey-Bass, 2000), 280–310.
14. "Manana," *Newsweek*, November 24, 1975, cited in Davis and Schoen, *Health and the War on Poverty*, 26.
15. Gomez, interviews.
16. Daniel Hawkins, interview by author, Washington, D.C., February 20, 2003.
17. Daniel Hawkins, communication to author, September 4, 2005.
18. Sister Angela Murdaugh, interview by author, Weslaco, Tex., March 11, 2003.
19. Stan Fisch and Nivia Fisch, interview by author, Harlingen, Tex., March 12, 2003, and subsequent communication.
20. Montejano, *Anglos and Mexicans*, 274–307.
21. Mel Huff, interview by author, Brownsville, Tex., March 11, 2003.
22. Ruben Edelstein, interview by author, Brownsville, Tex., March 11, 2003.
23. Gomez, interview; Basilio Hernandez, "Clinic Director Wants to Avoid Duplicating Work," *Brownsville Herald*, June 7, 1987.
24. Data reported by both centers in 2005 to Bureau of Primary Health Care, Health Resources and Services Administration, U.S. Department of Health and Human Services, Uniform Data System.
25. Emily Alpert, interview by author, Brownsville, Tex., March 11, 2003, and subsequent communications.
26. Kaiser Commission on Medicaid and the Uninsured, November 2005 Update.
27. Molly Ivins, television interview, *Now with Bill Moyers*, May 16, 2003.
28. Mel Huff, "Fight for Life: Couple Finds Care Just Out of Reach without Insurance Policy in Hand," *Brownsville Herald*, January 5, 2003; "Care Scarce for Uninsured," *Brownsville Herald*, January 6, 2003.
29. Number of centers in state from National Association of Community Health Centers, www.nachc.com, accessed December 2005.
30. Elena Marin, interview by author, Harlingen, Tex., March 14, 2003, and subsequent communication.
31. Project Digest prepared by Brownsville Community Health Center for Lower Rio Grande Valley Development Council, October 4, 2005. Cameron County population for 1960 from Geospatial and Statistical Data Center, University of Virginia Library, geostat@virginia.edu, accessed February 1, 2006.

32. Marin, interview.
33. Fernando del Valle, "Judge Appoints Su Clinica Receiver," *Valley Morning Star*, February 3, 2006.
34. Daniel Hawkins, communication to author, February 14, 2006.

Chapter 7. The Health Center Legacy

1. Daniel Hawkins, communication to author, September 4, 2005.
2. Donald Sykes, interview by author, Washington, D.C., August 31, 2004.
3. Finn, "Public Lives."
4. National Center for Health Statistics, *Health United States, 2005*, table 154.
5. Partridge, *APHSA Medicaid HEDIS Database Project*.
6. Falik et al., "Comparative Effectiveness of FQHCs."
7. Sardell, *U.S. Experiment in Social Medicine*, 156.
8. Bureau of Primary Health Care, Uniform Data System, http://bphc.hrsa.gov/uds/2004data/nattrend.htm, accessed November 30, 2005.
9. Mathematica Policy Research, Uninsured Patients in Community Health Centers, report for Bureau of Primary Health Care, Health Resources and Services Administration, 1999.
10. Michael K. Gusmano, Gerry Fairbrother, and Heidi Park, "Exploring the Limits of the Safety Net: Community Health Centers and Care for the Uninsured," *Health Affairs* 21, no. 6 (2002): 188–194.
11. Bureau of Primary Health Care, Uniform Data System, http://bphc.hrsa.gov/uds/2004data/nattrend.htm, accessed November 30, 2005.
12. Richard C. Bohrer, interview by author, Washington, D.C., August 31, 2005.
13. Sara Wilensky and Dylan H. Roby, "Health Centers and Health Insurance: Complements, Not Alternatives," *Journal of Ambulatory Care Management* 28, no. 4 (2005): 348–356.
14. Bureau of Primary Health Care, Uniform Data System, http://bphc.hrsa.gov/uds/2004data/nattrend.htm, accessed November 30, 2005.
15. Daniel R. Hawkins and Sara Rosenbaum, "The Challenges Facing Health Centers in a Changing Health Care System," in Stuart Altman, Uwe Reinhardt, and Alexandra Shields, eds., *The Future U.S. Health Care System: Who Will Care for the Poor and Uninsured* (Chicago: Health Administration Press, 1998), 99–122.
16. Kaiser Commission on Medicaid and the Uninsured, November 2005 Update.
17. Robert H. Frank, "The Income Gap Grows," *Philadelphia Inquirer*, November 27, 2005.
18. Robert D. Putnam, *Bowling Alone: The Collapse and Revival of American Community* (New York: Simon and Schuster, 2000).
19. Robert Putnam, "Bowling Together: The United State of America," *American Prospect*, February 11, 2002, 20–22.
20. Robert Pear, "Budget to Hurt Poor People on Medicaid, Report Says," *New York Times*, January 30, 2006.
21. Philip A. Klinkner with Rogers M. Smith, *The Unsteady March: The Rise and Decline of Racial Equality in America* (Chicago: University of Chicago Press, 1999).
22. Geiger, communication to author.
23. Boone, communication to author.
24. Gerard F. Anderson et al., "Health Spending in the United States and the Rest of the Industrialized World," *Health Affairs* 24, no. 4 (2005): 903–913.
25. Cynthia Smith et al., "National Health Spending in 2004: Recent Slowdown Led by Prescription Drug Spending," *Health Affairs* 25, no. 1 (2006): 186–196.

26. Ichiro Kawachi and Bruce P. Kennedy, *The Health of Nations: Why Inequality Is Harmful to Your Health* (New York: New Press, 2002).

27. National Center for Health Statistics, *Health United States, 2005*, table 23.

28. Ibid., table 25.

29. Van Coverden, interview.

30. Hatch, presentation at the W. K. Kellogg Symposium on Health of the Nation.

31. Geiger, communication to author, February 2005.

32. John Hatch, interview by author, Washington, D.C., June 7, 2006.

33. Sara Rosenbaum, communication to author, March 14, 2006.

34. Sykes, interview.

Alpert, Emily, operations director, Brownsville Community Health Center

Anderson, James (Andy), former medical director and cofounder, Jackson-Hinds Comprehensive Health Center

Barnes, Helen, chief of primary care–women's health, University Medical College Primary Care Clinic, Jackson Medical Mall; former maternal and child health director, Tufts-Delta Health Center

Barnwell, Thomas, former executive director, Beaufort-Jasper Comprehensive Health Services

Barron, Arnaldo, patient and former board member, William F. Ryan Community Health Center

Barros, Marsha (deceased), former board member, Roxbury Comprehensive Health Services and Massachusetts League of Community Health Centers

Bellber, Julio (Jay), president, RCHN Medical Foundation; former executive director, William F. Ryan Community Health Center

Blake, Tristram, executive director, South End Community Health Center

Bohrer, Richard, partner, Edward Martin & Associates, Inc.; former director, Division of Community and Migrant Health, Bureau of Primary Health Care, U.S. Department of Health and Human Services

Boone, Richard, former director, Research and Demonstrations, Community Action, Office of Economic Opportunity

Campbell, Emory, former director, Penn Center

Coleman, Thaddeous, former director of Environmental Services, Beaufort-Jasper-Hampton Comprehensive Health Services

Cradock, Jack, executive director, East Boston Neighborhood Health Center

Crawford, Anita, CEO, Roxbury Comprehensive Community Health Center

Driscoll, Daniel, executive director, Harbor Health Corporation; former director, Neponset Health Center

Dore, Louis, senior partner, Dore Law Firm; former director of Human Resources, Beaufort-Jasper-Hampton Comprehensive Health Services

Dorsey, L. C., professor of social work, Mississippi Valley State University; former executive director, Delta Health Center

Eddington, Sr. Trinita, director, St. Dominic's Community Clinic at Stewpot Community Services

Edelstein, Ruben, former mayor, city of Brownsville, Texas

Fisch, Nivia, certified nurse midwife, Harlingen Obstetrics and Gynecology Associates; former director, Su Clinica Familiar

Fisch, Stanley, physician, Harlingen Pediatrics Associates; former medical director, Su Clinica Familiar

Flores, Alix, project director, Campus Care Centers, Brownsville Community Health Center

Gardner, Roland, executive director, Beaufort-Jasper-Hampton Comprehensive Health Services

Geiger, H. Jack, professor emeritus, Arthur C. Logan Medical School, City University of New York; founding director of the first community health centers—Columbia Point, Boston, and Tufts-Delta Health Center, Mound Bayou, Mississippi

Gleason, Herbert P., former corporation counsel, Boston, and board chair, Health and Hospitals Department

Gomez, Paula, executive director, Brownsville Community Health Center; former staff member, Su Clinica Familiar

Gonzalez, Domingo, environmental activist; former organizer and board member, Su Clinica Familiar

Gottfried, Richard N., New York State assemblyman

Gruber, Kathy, director, Ryan/NENA Community Health Center

Hass, Gerald, medical director, South End Community Health Center

Hatch, John, professor emeritus of health behavior and health education, University of North Carolina School of Public Health; former director of development, Tufts-Delta Health Center

Hawkins, Daniel R., vice president for Federal, State, and Public Affairs, National Association of Community Health Centers; former executive director, Su Clinica Familiar

Hobson, William D., president and CEO, Watts Healthcare Corp.; former HEW staffer working with migrant health centers; former director, Bureau of Primary Health Care, U.S. Department of Health and Human Services

Holzberg, Harvey, president emeritus, Robert Wood Johnson Health System and Network; former executive director, Sunset Park Health Center

Hooley, James, former CEO, Neighborhood Health Plan of Massachusetts; organized early health centers for city of Boston

Huff, Mel, reporter, *Brownsville Herald*

Hunt, James W., president and CEO, Massachusetts League of Community Health Centers

Hunt, Jean, registered nurse and board member, Neponset Health Center

Kravitz, Sanford, former director, Research and Demonstrations and Training, Community Action, Office of Economic Opportunity

Krouser, Catherine, patient and former board member, William F. Ryan Community Health Center

Leifer, Jacqueline, senior partner, Feldesman, Tucker, Leifer and Fidell

Lowe, George, deputy director, Ryan/Chelsea-Clinton Community Health Center

Lugo, Maria, director, Patient Services, William F. Ryan Community Health Center

Maniece-Harrison, Bobbie, board chair, William F. Ryan Community Health Center

Marin, Elena, executive director and former medical director, Su Clinica Familiar

Minch, Barbra, president, William F. Ryan Community Health Center

Murdaugh, Sr. Angela, certified nurse midwife and director, Holy Family Birth Center

Murphy, Will, director, Outreach and Prevention, William F. Ryan Community Health Center

Raske, Kenneth, president, Greater New York Hospital Association

Salloway, Jeffrey, professor of health management and policy, University of New Hampshire; former postdoctoral fellow, Tufts Medical School, working with the first health centers

Scovell, Mel, former executive director, South End Community Health Center and Massachusetts League of Community Health Centers

Shirley, Aaron, associate professor of pediatrics, University of Mississippi Medical Center; developer and board member, Jackson Medical Mall Foundation; former executive director and cofounder, Jackson-Hinds Comprehensive Health Center

Shirley, Ollye, former chair, Jackson, Mississippi, Board of Education

Smith, Robert, executive director, Central Mississippi Health Services

Sykes, Donald, consultant; former director, Community Action Agency, Milwaukee, Wisconsin; director, Empowerment Zone Program, U.S. Department of Health and Human Services

Taylor, James, medical director, East Boston Neighborhood Health Center

Torrens, Paul, professor of health services, UCLA School of Public Health; first executive director, William F. Ryan Community Health Center

Van Coverden, Tom, president and CEO, National Association of Community Health Centers

Wessler, Judy, director, Commission on the Public's Health System, New York City

Woodard, Lathran, executive director, South Carolina Primary Health Care Association

Index

About the Author

Bonnie Lefkowitz grew up in and around Washington, D.C., and then spent fifteen years in New York City before moving back to the D.C. area. She spent her early career as a reporter for *Newsweek*, a medical writer, and a political activist. She served in the federal government for twenty-four years, developing health policy and supervising evaluation and research. As a "recovering bureaucrat," she writes about community health centers, care for low income and minority populations, and the social determinants of health. She holds a master's in public administration from the Kennedy School of Government at Harvard University, has published numerous articles and book chapters, and is the author of *Health Planning: Lessons for the Future* and coauthor of *Improving Health: It Doesn't Take a Revolution.*